Healing Fibromyalgia

The Three-Step Solution

David H. Trock, M.D.

Frances Chamberlain

BICENTENNIAL
1807
WILEY
2007
BICENTENNIAL

John Wiley & Sons, Inc.

Published by John Wiley & Sons, Inc., Hoboken, New Jersey
Published simultaneously in Canada

Wiley Bicentennial Logo: Richard J. Pacifico

Design and composition by Navta Associates, Inc.

The information contained in this book is not intended to serve as a replacement for professional medical advice. Any use of the information in this book is at the reader's discretion. The author and the publisher specifically disclaim any and all liability arising directly or indirectly from the use or application of any information contained in this book. A health care professional should be consulted regarding your specific situation.

For general information about our other products and services, please contact our Customer Care Department within the United States at (800) 762-2974, outside the United States at (317) 572-3993 or fax (317) 572-4002.

Wiley also publishes its books in a variety of electronic formats. Some content that appears in print may not be available in electronic books. For more information about Wiley products, visit our web site at www.wiley.com.

Library of Congress Cataloging-in-Publication Data:

Trock, David H.
    Healing fibromyalgia : the 3-step solution / David H. Trock, Frances Chamberlain.
       p. cm.
    Includes bibliographical references and index.
    ISBN 978-0-471-72428-5 (pbk.)
       1. Fibromyalgia—Popular works. I. Chamberlain, Frances. II. Title.
RC927.3.T7547 2007
616.7'4—dc22
2006032489

Printed in the United States of America

10 9 8 7 6 5 4 3 2 1

This book is dedicated to Elise, Amanda, and Daniel.

—David H. Trock, M.D.

I dedicate this book to my family for their support
during this long process of "birthing a book."

—Frances Chamberlain

In the face of uncertainty, there is nothing wrong with hope.

—BERNARD SIEGEL

CONTENTS

ACKNOWLEDGMENTS

Many thanks to our tireless agent Carole Abel, our wonderful editors Teryn Johnson and Christel Winkler, and the staff at John Wiley & Sons. We would especially like to acknowledge all the people with fibromyalgia who so willingly came forward to tell their stories.

Dr. Trock would also like to recognize the efforts of his devoted staff, particularly Anita Adzima and Janice Murner, the thoughtful leaders in the field of fibromyalgia, his colleagues at Danbury Hospital, and his wonderful patients who bravely endure.

Introduction

If you picked up this book looking for more ways to cope with fibromyalgia, you're in for a surprise. What we propose here is that fibromyalgia is not an incurable, chronic source of pain and misery but rather a temporary and reversible problem that can be fixed.

Just in the last year, a wealth of understanding has grown in the field, along with exciting and effective new therapies, many of which your doctor may be unaware. In addition, new medications have been approved to safely promote sleep and relieve pain in people with fibromyalgia. Physicians also have more insight about proper diet and holistic remedies, and inspiring technological advances have occurred that can revolutionize how fibromyalgia is treated in the future.

In this book you'll discover new diagnostic tools, like the functional magnetic resonance image (fMRI), which measures the body's response to pain; learn about studies proving that fibromyalgia is not a mystery disease but the result of an injury to the brain; and hear about treatments like **virtual reality therapy** and **repetitive transcranial magnetic stimulation (rTMS)**, medications such as **pregabalin and duloxetine**, and carefully selected over-the-counter supplements. The good news is that it is possible to recover. People with fibromyalgia are not doomed to a lifetime of suffering!

This may fly in the face of everything you've ever heard before, and it certainly is a new way to look at things; however, remarkable advances in research have provided a realistic path to recovery.

We now know that fibromyalgia falls into three categories—postinjury (including posterior neck compression), postillness, and stress driven. Once you discover the source of your fibromyalgia, you will have a better understanding of the syndrome. A whole new range of treatments and medications will help you to cope with pain and discomfort, and you can develop a plan for recovery.

The days of a doctor writing a quick prescription to treat fibromyalgia symptoms are fading fast. Doctors are working in conjunction with holistic practitioners, and the Internet has become a source of information and education for anyone interested in the neurobiology of pain and stress. As a result, people are more knowledgeable when they visit their doctors' offices and can be active participants in producing successful outcomes.

In the United States, where a woman's life span has been extended to roughly eighty years, it is unacceptable that fibromyalgia still causes so much suffering. Given the demographics of everyone who is affected—five million people in the United States, mostly women between twenty and fifty years of age—fibromyalgia should be a national issue that attracts the same degree of funding as other highly prevalent conditions. The time has come to put fibromyalgia on the same short list of priorities.

When we consider these five million fibromyalgia sufferers, many of them women in their childbearing years, it's easy to imagine the exponential impact on others around them. People with fibromyalgia may be unable to care for children, have normal relationships with their spouses, or be as productive as they would like in the workplace. The emotional and financial toll is mind numbing. Fibromyalgia is a true hardship for millions of men, women, and children, and it is obviously time to take the condition seriously.

It will take a grassroots effort to ensure that government agencies and insurance companies cover the expense of treating fibromyalgia. Although the fibromyalgia solution presented herein is relatively inexpensive for some people, others may require novel medications or costly diagnostic tools that aren't covered under most health plans.

Fibromyalgia sufferers must also have access to and coverage for nonpharmaceutical treatments. Massage therapy, proper psychological support, and alternative pain-management techniques are just some of the basic types of complementary care that people should be able to receive. The economic consequences of fibromyalgia—unemployment, disability payments, and worker's compensation—clearly demand our attention, and the expense of proper care will ultimately be money well spent.

The support of families and friends is extremely important in a person's recovery from fibromyalgia. You don't exist in a vacuum, and you won't get better in one, either. Spouses, children, parents, and significant friends must become educated about fibromyalgia and must learn to support their loved ones. A lack of understanding, empathy, or compassion on the part of friends and family can be detrimental when dealing with such a complicated syndrome that develops from a variety of factors. If you are a fibromyalgia sufferer, try to educate people around you. If you picked up this book because you know someone with fibromyalgia and want to support that person, read on and learn all that you can. Women sometimes find themselves not being taken seriously or not being believed because fibromyalgia was, in the past, dismissed as a woman's illness, and because there hasn't been one specific course of treatment.

People with fibromyalgia have more options now than ever before. From this book, they'll gain a better understanding of what may have caused them to develop fibromyalgia, whether an accident, illness, or trauma. They'll also learn about various types of pain generators and look at treatment options. Understanding their symptoms and which of these might overlap with other conditions will help them to recover.

Part I of this book explains exactly what fibromyalgia is, and part II will help you to chart the course of recovery. Each step you take will bring new information, debate, and controversy. The path will be slightly different for each individual, just as the symptoms have varied, but the time has come to embrace new ideas, discuss the possibilities, and explore the realistic goal of complete recovery.

PART I

The Problem

1

Fibromyalgia and Its Common Triggers

Fibromyalgia is a syndrome of widespread pain and fatigue. Its underlying causes are many, although in each case the symptoms appear to be driven by injury to the central nervous system. The initial injury may appear obvious at first, like a car accident or a sudden illness, but sometimes the inciting event is more insidious, such as an emotional trauma that occurred months or even years before the onset of fibromyalgia. In some cases, the trauma to the central nervous system isn't a single event but a constant barrage of daily unhealthy stress. While the precipitating factors are too numerous to mention, the symptoms are strangely alike—fatigue and diffuse pain. Overlapping conditions such as irritable bowel syndrome, migraine headaches, and insomnia are also common, and a heightened awareness of external stimuli (stress, painful touch, loud noise, noxious smells, and bright lights) appears to arise from a phenomenon known as **central sensitivity**.

Fibromyalgia has been a puzzling syndrome ever since it was described as neurasthenia more than a hundred years ago by Sir William Osler:

> Neurasthenia appears to be the expression of a morbid, unhealthy reaction to stimuli acting on the nervous centers that preside over the functions of organic life. Sleeplessness is a frequent concomitant and may be the first manifestation, and when the spinal symptoms predominate, the patient complains of weariness on the least exertion. The aching pain in the back or in the back of the neck is the most constant complaint in these cases. Occasionally, there may be disturbances of sensation, particularly a feeling of numbness and tingling.

A century later, we still don't know exactly why someone gets fibromyalgia, but we are now able to document and understand the subtle changes that occur inside the nervous system. Advanced medical technology can identify the hidden abnormalities inside the brain of a fibromyalgia sufferer by using functional magnetic resonance image (fMRI) scanning. We can measure pain messengers such as **substance P** in the **cerebrospinal fluid** and can even track neurotransmitters and the signals that they carry from the brain to various parts of the body. These advances allow us not only to understand, but to measure, someone's sensitivity and reaction to pain and to clarify that fibromyalgia is not a subjective disorder but instead is quantifiable pain and discomfort directly related to an injury to the central nervous system. We have a clearer picture of how certain illnesses and trauma (physical or emotional) can trigger fibromyalgia in a susceptible person. For example, it is now accepted that there is an association between fibromyalgia and other conditions such as **whiplash**, post-Lyme syndrome, and **systemic lupus erythematosus**. The connection to these conditions is an important discovery. For many years, people with fibromyalgia suffered without having a clue as to why they might have this syndrome. Now doctors are able to evaluate a patient's medical history and come up with a logical explanation for the symptoms. It's a tremendous relief to find a contributing factor because knowing the root of the symptoms can help to determine a plan of action.

An Injury to the Central Nervous System

If you've been diagnosed with fibromyalgia, you probably wonder why this has happened to you. The answer, as far as scientists can determine, lies not in the peripheral muscles and joints where most of the pain is felt but in the delicate cervical spine or in the *brain itself*, where the message of pain is both received and interpreted. Whether the damage arises from a single event or cumulative traumas, infection to the brain, or chronic emotional stress is unclear, but the brain is susceptible to damage from many assaults that are not always obvious.

In fibromyalgia, injuries inside the brain initially involve three areas: the **limbic system**, the **hippocampus**, and the **hypothalamus**.

The limbic system is the most primitive center of the brain, from which feelings of suffering and stress emerge. The hippocampus is a sensitive area of the brain in which memory is stored. It is highly vulnerable to trauma and chronic stress, and it ultimately affects one's learned behavior and response to emotional triggers. The hypothalamus is the master thermostat of the brain, where the automatic functions of the body are regulated; these include arousal, blood flow, body temperature, and hormonal balance.

The Hippocampus

The hippocampus is the part of the brain in which memories are stored. It is quite sensitive to trauma and, in fact, has been seen to atrophy, or shrink, when an individual endures too much stress. This can occur in the brain of a person who has suffered a childhood trauma or long periods of depression. Furthermore, the hippocampus can secrete substance P (a pain messenger) under such circumstances, thereby sensitizing people with post-traumatic stress to more physical pain. It is no surprise that for someone who suffers from fibromyalgia and dormant memories of stress, the condition of the delicate hippocampus may contribute to how that person perceives pain and responds to it.

The **hypothalamic-pituitary-adrenal axis (HPA axis)** helps to regulate the body's response to stress, partly by controlling one's level of **cortisol**. Brief periods of stress increase the level of cortisol, which produces the protective fight-or-flight response, but chronic stress is unhealthy and adversely affects the delicate balance of the brain and the body. We all deal with a certain amount of stress in our lives. This can be as simple as slamming on the brakes to avoid an accident or rushing to make an appointment on time. There are also other stressors that aren't momentary and don't seem to go away. Perhaps you are coping with a difficult relationship, a job where you can't keep up with demands, or a busy family life. If a situation is stressful enough to cause your body to keep producing cortisol at unhealthy levels, there are physical consequences.

Stress hormones—in particular, cortisol—can cause the atrophy of parts of the brain. Stress hormones originate in the hypothalamus, the center of the brain, and when everything is working properly, our bodies produce the right amount of cortisol. It is when the stress never seems to end that cortisol production increases to the point where the brain is affected.

Feedback in the brain works to keep cortisol production within normal bounds, but during periods of stress or illness, the HPA axis provides a temporary increase of cortisol production. This increase occurs because of the body's natural reaction to stress, but in the case of fibromyalgia, lengthy periods of chronic stress cause a dysregulation of the system and a failure to respond properly to trauma or illness.

For example, Patricia, age forty-five, is a hardworking school administrator who has raised three children. Ten years ago, she suffered a neck injury. Then, everything seemed to change. She had not only pain in the back of the neck but diffuse muscular tender points, one of the key symptoms of fibromyalgia. She struggled with exhaustion and fatigue and had diffi-

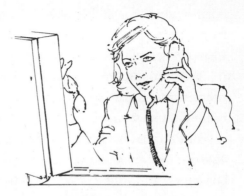

Chronic daily stress causes an unhealthy imbalance of the mind and body. Energy, sleep, pain perception, and immune function are all affected.

culty sleeping, muscle tightness, and an aching, irritable bladder. She couldn't concentrate. "It was like I never got any relief; I never felt totally like myself after that initial injury," she said. The demands of her job and her children and the day-to-day responsibilities of a household became impossible to manage. Fortunately, her husband was willing and able to shoulder some of these duties, but even so, picking up her youngest child became an excruciating task. Some days, plagued by cystitis, headaches, and muscle pain, she just wanted to stay in bed in a darkened room.

For any woman who has dealt with the multiple demands of children, household, and work, it's clear that there are few avenues of escape. Even if she can't drag herself out of bed, the household comes to her. Patricia struggled through day after day. Some periods were manageable, others intolerable. The whole family had to make compromises because of her fibromyalgia.

Her recovery took nearly a year, but the time went quickly, and now she almost feels like her normal self again. After a careful medical assessment, it was discovered that Patricia had been suffering from a protracted myofascial pain syndrome and a sleep disorder, both of which fueled her fibromyalgia. She received integrative care from a rheumatologist and a holistic practitioner. A combination of manual therapy designed to relax her muscles, along with guided imagery, an adjustment to her diet, and a short course of a novel **membrane-stabilizing medication** was orchestrated for her, and the results were good.

For Patricia, having a name for all the disparate aches and pains, as well as a plan of action for treatment, "was like getting a second chance at life." She learned not to push too hard and overextend herself. Prioritizing and doing what needed to be done first meant that she could stop and rest without feeling guilty. It took time, but it was worth it.

The bottom line is that fibromyalgia affects a person's ability to function. The individual not only develops aches and pains but may also report difficulty coping with the demands of daily living. The person typically struggles to keep up at work and needs more time to recuperate after ordinary exertion. People with fibromyalgia often become concerned because their symptoms mirror certain potentially serious diseases, so they visit their primary-care physicians to be evaluated. Indeed, a medical workup is a reasonable thing to get because it is essential to rule out other conditions that mimic fibromyalgia, for which proper treatment might be different. This important point will be discussed later in the book. It suffices to say that your fibromyalgia might be triggered by a persistent pain generator due to previous trauma or a precipitating illness. Once this trigger is established, the focus should quickly return to an appropriate plan of action for fibromyalgia. It's helpful to address the precipitating factor—illness, injury, or trauma—and not to expect one strategy to resolve all symptoms. Reactive fibromyalgia, the fibromyalgia that occurs after sudden physical trauma, can be particularly difficult to treat and needs to be identified right away. Any lengthy delay can be detrimental to recovery because living with fibromyalgia for a long period of time, without addressing it, leads only to increased levels of stress, pain, and frustration for the person involved and further establishes the problem of central sensitivity.

During the diagnostic process, be as specific about your symptoms as possible. Many people complain of fatigue, but fatigue means different things to everyone, and it can indicate a variety of conditions. In fibromyalgia, people complain about being physically tired, mentally exhausted, or simply unable to stay awake. This might be very different from someone who has daytime drowsiness but otherwise has energy to complete tasks, or from the person who has muscular aches but no tiredness. Articulate your symptoms clearly—this is no time to be vague or to minimize the way you feel. Tell it like it really is, even if it's slightly embarrassing to admit that you sometimes fall asleep at your desk when no one else is around or nap at the wheel of your car before the kids get out of school. Any specific details that you can add will help your physician understand the extent of your physical and mental exhaustion. In addition, with fibromyalgia there is often widespread musculoskeletal pain, sensitivity to touch, and an absence of objective swelling. Because all of these symptoms can overlap with many other conditions, help your doctor to rule out everything else and then get down to the business of treating the fibromyalgia.

An accurate diagnosis might take some time, so it's crucial that people with fibromyalgia have the support of their families from the very beginning. Obviously, this is easier said than done. One husband of a fibromyalgia sufferer admitted that because his wife wasn't diagnosed for several years, he often found himself wondering whether she was just a hypochondriac. "The syndrome is unpredictable," he said. "So, you ascribe certain circumstances to each flare-up, such as, she was hungry or she was too tired. Then it becomes a question of whether she did something to bring on the symptoms, or maybe it was my fault. I can't imagine how a child would react to this because it's so difficult for adults. I think a child would always be feeling guilty, like Mommy was sick because he was naughty. It's not a simple thing to live with."

Caroline, age forty-two, is another woman whose life was nearly ruined by fibromyalgia. She is single and doesn't have children. Her life is perhaps somewhat different from Patricia's. She hasn't ever been particularly sick. She did, however, have a traffic accident four years ago when she was hit from behind at a stoplight. Her injuries, whiplash and a broken wrist, healed with time, but suddenly, out of nowhere, she began to suffer from extreme pain. It wasn't in the joints or necessarily related to the whiplash and the broken wrist, but the pain was always there, in a dozen different places. She spent sleepless nights, struggled through days with headaches and irritable bowel syndrome, and began to miss more and more days of work. She became depressed, as one might expect, and heard once too often that all these symptoms might be related to her depression. Often, it can be difficult to determine whether depression is just another symptom of the fibromyalgia, or whether it's a result of the pain and the compromised lifestyle. Certainly, it was a struggle for Caroline to keep her spirits up when she could barely accomplish daily tasks, especially when people didn't believe there was anything wrong with her. Even without the added burden of a family, Caroline struggled through her workday. Only when she received a diagnosis and instructions to take time off work to begin her recovery did things began to change. She needed to concentrate on herself, exploring all the treatment options and most especially taking time to rest, before her symptoms eased. Like Patricia, Caroline waited too long to find out what was wrong. Because she had lived with fibromyalgia for many months before her diagnosis, her recovery required a careful unraveling of symptoms. When she understood what had triggered her illness and which factors made it worse, she could begin to get better.

One key to diagnosing fibromyalgia is searching for **tender points**—specific areas that are particularly sensitive to pressure—mostly around the neck and the lower back. The pain can be anywhere and everywhere, although it seems to concentrate in specific locations that are predictable among fibromyalgia sufferers.

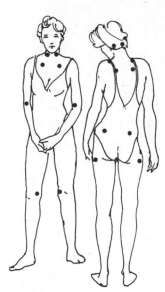

A good physician can diagnose fibromyalgia by finding a majority of the eighteen tender points illustrated. The tender points are found in a symmetrical fashion, both above and below the waist. Basically, tender points are the sensitive spots at the centers of certain muscles and in certain places where muscles join tendons. A caregiver can apply pressure to each point and observe the individual's pain reaction. Note that these tender points are not just tender; they are definitely *painful*. The pain is generally in the muscles, the ligaments, and the tendons, and some people say that they ache all over. Others say that

Most fibromyalgia sufferers have a majority of the eighteen tender points in a symmetrical pattern above and below the waist.

it feels as if the muscles have been overworked or strained. It's also not uncommon for people to have the burning and tingling pain of neuropathy. Needless to say, if a physician presses a patient's tender point, a spot where muscles are aching and throbbing or sending out shooting, stabbing pains, the patient will react dramatically. If the patient has a sufficient number of tender points, and a thorough workup suggests no other cause, then fibromyalgia is likely to be the diagnosis.

The muscles around the neck, shoulders, chest and rib cage, lower back, and hips are inclined to be most painful in fibromyalgia. It's the diffuse nature of muscular pain—the way it is spread

---

Functional Magnetic Resonance Image Scanning

A novel approach to mapping a pain message in the brain is with functional MRI scanning (fMRI). The standard MRI and fMRI have overlapping methods of operating, but the main difference is of mapping anatomy versus physiology. While the standard MRI gives a bird's-eye view of anatomical abnormalities such as a brain tumor, a stroke, a bleed, atrophy, and so on, the fMRI basically looks at where the blood is flowing. This is accomplished by mapping where the oxygen is from one second to the next.

For example, if you produce a source of pain in a person's left foot, a standard brain MRI would be unchanged, but the fMRI would reflect increased blood flow in the right sensory cortex. Using the fMRI on people with fibromyalgia has demonstrated important differences in blood flow through several parts of the brain, particularly the limbic system, which controls, in part, the degree of suffering perceived by the person. It should be mentioned, however, that fMRI isn't a perfect tool; it's still considered experimental and is rarely covered by insurance plans. In addition, how the radiologist reads the results can vary significantly. What it does offer, though, is the possibility of a new objective measure of pain perception in people with fibromyalgia, something that will help to validate the complaints of those who suffer.

throughout the body—that distinguishes fibromyalgia from other regional pain syndromes such as **myofascial pain**, which typically affects only one quadrant of the body. Keep in mind, however, that the two conditions—fibromyalgia and myofascial pain—frequently coexist, particularly after whiplash or other such traumas.

While a large percentage of people who have fibromyalgia are women of childbearing age, any individual can get it, including children. Men get fibromyalgia, too, although they are less likely to see a doctor about it. Moreover, doctors tend not to make the diagnosis in men, in some cases due to gender bias. Men generally have fewer symptoms, and these may be less severe; however, a man with fibromyalgia is still in significantly more pain and discomfort than is a man *without* fibromyalgia. Much of what is written in *Healing Fibromyalgia* will be useful to men as well. A man with fibromyalgia may find it more difficult to locate a physician who believes this is the correct diagnosis, though, because fibromyalgia is considered a woman's illness. This can be isolating and troubling to the male patient. It's the reverse of the gender discrimination practiced against women who have chest pain; until recently, heart attacks had always been considered a man's problem. Clearly, this isn't the case, and the gender bias is unfair. There are resources for men with fibromyalgia, just as there are for women with chest pain, and it will be the persistent man who can go against societal expectations and work to solve his difficulties with fibromyalgia.

One man who succeeded at this was Jack. As a truck driver, he had experienced a particularly severe low back injury, followed by diffuse muscular pain that kept him out of work for months. He grew depressed and slept poorly, began to drink more, and gained weight. After the fibromyalgia diagnosis and the lengthy process of applying for temporary disability, he sought counseling, started taking antidepressant medication, and stopped drinking. He began a light aerobic exercise regimen, eventually lost the weight he gained, and noticed an improvement in his sleeping patterns. He found tremendous relief by using electrical muscle stimulation on the affected areas of his back. This technique of allowing gentle electrical currents to massage deep into the affected tissue is particularly successful in both physical therapy and chiropractic. Once Jack was trained to use the equipment and had it available at home, he discovered that he could achieve relief from his symptoms. He continues with physical therapy, rests when he needs to, and uses **transcutaneous electrical nerve stimulation (TENS)** for immediate relief when his symptoms are painful. Best of all, he's back at work, nearly full time, feeling productive once more.

In older people, the diagnosis of fibromyalgia is often delayed because the symptoms of pain and fatigue occur in conjunction with other chronic conditions such as degenerative disk disease and arthritis of the spine. The physician may also suspect depression or malignancy as a root cause. Occasionally, a patient who already has a clear diagnosis of **lupus, Lyme disease,** or chronic rheumatic condition will also present with fibromyalgia. Sadly, these conditions are not mutually exclusive; in fact, there seems to be a higher incidence of fibromyalgia among people who already have an underlying rheumatic disease. We'll examine the connection between fibromyalgia and other conditions in later chapters.

Like Caroline and Patricia, whose problems were described earlier, you might have started out with a few minor aches and pains before those developed into a pattern of diffuse, debilitating muscular soreness. Like these women, you may have trouble sleeping or may suffer from fatigue, anxiety, or depression. Perhaps it's getting harder to perform optimally at your job or keep up with the chores at home, your family, your social life, and other activities and interests. You and your doctor might already have ruled out a host of serious illnesses—things you don't have—and finally arrived at the diagnosis of fibromyalgia. If you don't necessarily feel grateful that it's fibromyalgia, hopefully the knowledge that it isn't something worse has given you cause for optimism.

We are closer than ever to understanding the problem; according to most of the cutting-edge research, it appears that fibromyalgia is triggered by an injury to the central nervous system. The initial insult might be a form of physical trauma such as a car accident (particularly, whiplash), an infection such as Lyme disease or hepatitis C, or one of many different kinds of emotional upheaval, such as bereavement, assault, or the repressed fallout from childhood abuse. Some cases do not result from any single event but only from the chronic daily stress of the modern world. Examples of this include job dissatisfaction, a malevolent boss, and spousal abuse (verbal or physical), among other forms of discord.

We've all probably dealt with difficult work situations. Imagine for a moment, or just remember, what it is like to work for someone who disapproves of everything you do. You can't afford to quit, at least not until you have another job prospect, so you go in to work, day after day, knowing that the boss will belittle you, yell at you, leave nasty notes on your desk, reprimand you for taking too much time at lunch, and generally make your life miserable. The mounting stress of such a situation leads to anxiety that you take home at night. Perhaps you become less able to cope with other stressors in your life or have bad dreams that interrupt your sleep. The chronic nature of this stress leads to the overproduction of cortisol, which we mentioned earlier in this chapter, and you become ever vigilant and hyperaware, always watching for the next attack from this malevolent boss.

Any stress that you feel at work, under such unfavorable circumstances, extends beyond nine to five. You may not sleep as well, may have bad dreams, or may feel anxious when you're not at work. Some people are better than others at leaving work where it belongs, but lots of people carry this stress home, in unnael in ways, and it has a negative impact that they don't anticipate. If you have fibromyalgia and your work situation is particularly negative, look at techniques to address this source of stress in your life, perhaps before or at least simultaneously with your recovery.

In certain cases, we keep dormant issues hidden even from ourselves, which can interfere with our peace of mind or a good night's sleep. This is just one aspect of **post-traumatic stress disorder (PTSD)** that will receive attention when we discuss the biology of stress later in the book. PTSD may result from a situation such as childhood abuse or from living with the constant threat of violence. Perhaps you have long since forgotten about repeated episodes of abuse—it's not uncommon for people to block out these memories, to some degree. Yet even if you don't remember the initial trauma anymore, that doesn't mean it is resolved.

When we bring up childhood abuse, you might think of violent or physically abusive situations. PTSD can also result from less obvious forms of abuse. Perhaps a young girl was left alone at home, long before she was ready for that responsibility. She became fearful of cars driving by, anticipated someone knocking at the door, and was agitated by any unexplained noises in the house. Underneath these superficial fears lurked a very real dread that her parents might not come home. She experienced feelings of abandonment and despair every time they left after dark. Today she is an adult woman, but being alone in a dark house triggers anxiety that she can't explain. Fear and sadness stem from early childhood experiences that she has dismissed as unimportant. True, other children might have similar experiences and might emerge into adulthood unscarred, but this particular woman now suffers from PTSD symptoms that she doesn't trace back to this childhood situation until she undertakes therapy and a little soul searching.

The Stage Is Set

Even in a healthy, stable body, many things can trigger brief periods of insomnia, a heightened sensitivity to pain, and other symptoms of fibromyalgia. If you have a family history of fibromyalgia, particularly a mother or a sister with the syndrome, your odds of developing fibromyalgia are higher. Tests have shown that female relatives of people with fibromyalgia have a heightened sensitivity to pain. In some cases, low levels of **corticotropin-releasing hormone (CRH)** indicate a predisposition to post-traumatic stress disorder, a precursor to fibromyalgia. There may also be a link between fibromyalgia and eating disorders, particularly in obese people with insomnia.

How Pain Generators Work

Physical abnormalities, such as degenerative disk disease or other forms of arthritis, can serve as chronic **pain generators** and can perpetuate fibromyalgia. Whiplash is a particularly troubling source of fibromyalgia, as is an episode of Lyme disease. People with systemic lupus are also more likely to develop fibromyalgia, and since many of the features of fibromyalgia overlap with chronic fatigue syndrome, it's not unusual for the two conditions to coexist.

The diagnosis of fibromyalgia is not always so clear-cut. One person might suffer through an illness or an injury, then might recover, return to work, and suddenly come down with symptoms of fibromyalgia. There isn't always an obvious correlation between one event and another. Even more puzzling, perhaps, is when fibromyalgia comes along many years after a trauma, making it difficult for the person to connect what might have happened in the distant past with what is going on medically today. Women or men who were victims of childhood sexual abuse or other childhood traumas are sometimes unaware of the lingering impact that their traumas may have on their sleep or sense of well-being. They may still be susceptible to getting fibromyalgia if they have not resolved these issues.

Some people need to confront their abusers and extract apologies. Others might achieve resolution by remembering the incidents, discussing them with their therapists, finding a way to forgive or forget, and resolving to move on with their lives. Repressing feelings of anger or humiliation that might linger for years afterward only contributes to chronic stress. Searching your past for experiences that were particularly stressful or troubling, and then working in a systematic way to resolve those experiences, will help you to lead a healthier life in the future.

Sometimes a person has a healthy, normal lifestyle when an injury or an inciting event unmasks a dormant issue. Maybe there is a reunion with an abuser or a new situation triggers emotions similar to those experienced in a previous trauma. Shortly afterward, tender points, fatigue, sleeplessness, and depression occur. It is particularly vexing when there doesn't appear to be any precipitating factor for these symptoms, and medical tests fail to pinpoint specific conditions. When this occurs, people become victims a second time when they are not taken seriously.

Consider the case of Janet. She occasionally recalls memories of an uncle who insisted on taking her for car rides, alone. As an adult, she knows that he was sexually abusive to her, but the actual incidents remain unresolved. There was never a confrontation, a confession, or any kind of resolution. It's just an emotional burden she carries with her. When she developed fibromyalgia, she became especially limited by lower-back pain, fatigue, and sleeplessness. Nothing seemed to ease her suffering. She made no conscious connection between her troubled past and her poor health today.

In fact, her efforts to recover focused almost exclusively on treating muscle soreness and back pain. She relied on analgesics and muscle relaxants to relieve the pain, she cut back her activities and hours of work, and she limited household chores and family activities. In short, she compromised the fullness of her life because she didn't make a connection between her past emotional trauma and her present pain.

In her case, it was imperative to go back to the root of her distress and work through the emotional scars; then she could address her physical symptoms.

Tapering off medications, along with starting a regimen of gentle stretching, weight loss, and a careful diet, under the supervision of her physician, helped her to get back her life after years of suffering.

It's important to remember that many people with fibromyalgia have never been the victims of sexual abuse. Moreover, the majority of victims of childhood sexual abuse will never develop fibromyalgia. Yet early childhood abuse has been shown to have lasting effects on brain neurobiology, and it is one of the more insidious causes of PTSD that can predispose a person to fibromyalgia. Two sisters, exposed to the same stressors, might reach adulthood and one will have fibromyalgia, while the other will not. Although there are some familial tendencies in fibromyalgia, it's not clear why one woman with a history of childhood abuse will develop this syndrome, while another won't. What we do know is that the abuse has an impact on the brain, predisposing a person to develop PTSD and later, perhaps, fibromyalgia. This fertile area of psychosomatic medicine will be covered in the next chapter.

The Impact of Stress

The ordinary rigors of daily life come into play as well. Someone may live with a particularly difficult burden that he or she cannot discuss with others, so this person soldiers on and accepts the daily pain. It's hard to quantify the impact this may have on an individual, but it's fair to say that chronic stress is unhealthy, has a deleterious effect on the immune system, contributes to insomnia, and can trigger fibromyalgia.

Here is an illustration of the impact of daily stress. Dorothea's husband is unpredictable. Some days he might fly into a rage because the lawnmower doesn't work or he doesn't like what Dorothea bought at the grocery store. She tries to anticipate his needs and wants. She protects him from bad news, if possible, such as a high electric bill or something one of the children has done that he won't like. Yet the constant worrying about what might trigger his temper tantrums and all the energy involved in keeping his life stress free means that Dorothea lives in a state of continual anxiety. Similar to a boss who has a vendetta against you, an angry, unreasonable spouse can make his or her mark in very unhealthy ways.

Dorothea didn't feel the impact of his unreasonable rage only on occasional bad days. It was a daily, cumulative effect because she always anticipated trouble and never wanted to be caught off guard. Her actions became almost unconscious, filtering out anything that might annoy him—such as the barking dog, a ringing phone, or quarrelling children. After some months, she realized that she couldn't fall asleep at night because her whole body was tense. Then, she had periods of wakefulness during the night and sometimes woke long before dawn. The fatigue lessened her ability to cope with the normal stressors in her own life. She felt exhausted all the time and suffered from severe headaches, intermittent cystitis, and irritable bowels. When her physician explained the relevance of the tender points in conjunction with all the other symptoms, Dorothea understood what was going on. Getting better, for her, had to start with the root of the problem—a difficult relationship that needed a lot of work.

If you have experienced the symptoms of fibromyalgia but can't relate them to any specific illness or trauma, you must search to discover the cause and figure out why you were susceptible in the first place. Healing begins when you address critical issues that are causing you stress and anxiety, whether they occurred years ago or are now part of your daily life.

The symptoms of fibromyalgia remain strikingly similar in most people, although it's crucial to remember that in each case, fibromyalgia develops as a result of emotional or physical trauma. The term *trauma* does not necessarily mean a life-threatening accident. The initial injury can be very subtle and the immediate damage may be overlooked, but the consequences of central sensitivity eventually become apparent. Something happened to the brain—the central nervous system—even if you are not aware of it. If you were in a minor car accident, you might have had a silent whiplash injury or an insidious concussion. If you endured an emotional trauma from which you feel that you've recovered, the damage may have been suppressed, but it didn't necessarily go away. In each case, the delicate mind-body balance has been upset.

Before we go any further, it's important that we describe the symptoms of fibromyalgia. If you have already been diagnosed, you know only too well what they are, but if you are still struggling to find out exactly what is going on, this list may help you to understand the syndrome. We'll go into each symptom in greater detail later in the book.

First of all, most fibromyalgia sufferers complain of pain. It can be aching, throbbing pain or intense, burning pain, generally with tender points in symmetrical locations throughout the body. Many people feel fatigue, and, again, the intensity can vary from person to person. Some people may cope with it, while others find that the fatigue drains them of every ounce of energy. Sleep disorders, the inability to achieve full, restful sleep, are a hallmark symptom. In addition, many people suffer from irritable bowel syndrome—constipation, diarrhea, frequent abdominal pain, and other gastrointestinal complaints. There are chronic headaches, **TMJ (temporomandibular joint**; jaw-related face or head pain), and then, to a lesser extent, cognitive or memory impairment, irritable bladder, dry eyes and mouth, dizziness, or a heightened sensitivity to bright lights or noise.

A good physician should be able to determine whether the imbalance in the central nervous system is due to a lingering physical injury, an insidious sleep disturbance, a chronic illness, or an emotional issue that can overlap with any of these. This is an arduous task, even by modern standards. It takes patience, understanding, and a healthy partnership between patient and caregiver.

Fortunately, recent research has taken much of the mystery out of fibromyalgia. If a disruption of the delicate mind-body balance has occurred due to trauma or insult, healing can take place. To suffer needlessly from fibromyalgia is unacceptable because the human body, in the absence of permanent damage and with the proper care and treatment, should be able to recover—or "reboot," if you will. The key to recovery is an accurate diagnosis and a determination of the type of fibromyalgia that you have. It's important to know the precipitating factor and the existence of stubborn pain generators before you begin treatment. As you'll see in the following chapters, fibromyalgia is unique. No one person has the same experience as someone else, although there may be many similarities. Talking to other fibromyalgia sufferers may help you to learn to cope with your own ailments. Finally, once you understand what caused the syndrome and have sorted out which symptoms are a result of fibromyalgia, this book will help you to create a plan that allows you to climb out of the depths. Subsequent chapters of *Healing Fibromyalgia* will take you step by step from the onset of the syndrome through diagnosis and treatment and, most important, to a healthy recovery.

2

The Biology of Chronic Stress

There is a tendency to blame fibromyalgia on anxiety, depression, and insomnia, as if these things actually caused the illness. The reality, however, is that these things do not cause fibromyalgia but are symptoms of the larger problem of central sensitivity. Indeed, it is more likely that central sensitivity—the imbalance within the central nervous system that misinterprets normal touch as tenderness—is also responsible for alterations of mood and energy and many other symptoms of fibromyalgia.

This chapter explains how prolonged exposure to stress sets up conditions for the development of fibromyalgia. With a better understanding of the sensitive areas inside the brain and the substances they produce, we can comprehend the symptoms that arise from central sensitivity and therefore learn how to treat them better.

Back to Basics

To help you recognize that fibromyalgia is not a primary disorder of the muscles and joints but a temporary injury to the central nervous system, let's look at the brain structures involved and the **neurotransmitters** produced by them. This is one of the most important aspects of understanding the syndrome. Those painful muscles and tendons are not permanently damaged but are responding to changes inside the CNS.

For starters, the essential rule inside the nervous system is that **neurons** need a contrast of charges in order to function. Neurons generate **ions** within their cell membranes to create a resting potential, and they release ions across their cell membranes to create an action potential. The release of neurotransmitters across gates and channels of a neuron delivers a message to a neighboring neuron, whereas a **hormone** delivers a message through the bloodstream to a distant receptor.

Neurotransmitters are made of small building blocks of **amino acids** or **lipids**, which are constantly manufactured and recycled to serve as chemical messengers. Their unique receptors are designed to receive messages that are either excitatory or inhibitory. It's not unusual for two or more messages to converge and cancel each other out. The slightest alteration of the structure, amount, or availability of neurotransmitters can have a profound effect on our brain chemistry (mood, energy, creativity, pain interpretation, hormone release, etc.). And while there are trillions of possible messages in the brain at any given time, we require only a few hundred neurotransmitters in various combinations to make us who we are. Think of this as being analogous to having only twenty-six letters in the English alphabet available to create a multitude of words. Among the many circulating neurotransmitters, those listed as follows are the major players affecting fibromyalgia.

NEUROTRANSMITTERS THAT AFFECT PAIN

Excitatory	*Inhibitory*	*Regulatory*
Substance P	**Endorphins**	Cortisol
Glutamate	**Gamma-amino-butyric acid (GABA)**	**Norepinephrine**
Aspartate/N-methyl-D-aspartate (NMDA)	Serotonin	Acetylcholine
Nerve growth factor	**Dopamine**	Growth hormone

A sudden emotional stress will activate the primitive and protective fight-or-flight response that's designed to rev us up and get us out of danger. An unhealthy level of sustained emotional stress, however, can lead to a dampening of the normal regulatory systems and predisposes us to the early features of fibromyalgia, such as anxiety, insomnia, muscle tension, and headache. This alteration in the brain's protective mechanism is the driving force behind post-traumatic stress: a subconscious foot on the gas pedal, if you will.

So, how does a constant stream of stress or a bad memory you can't forget affect your perception of body pain? The answer is complicated and begins with a concept known as **long-term potentiation (LTP)**. In a nutshell, the accumulation of literally millions of messages is required for complex thinking or activity. This develops in infancy when the simplest task requires neurons to stimulate the dendrites, or message centers, of other neurons until a desired action is achieved. Then the resulting message is transmitted to the brain's higher centers to successfully complete the task. Examples include reaching for an object or crying when you're hungry. Not surprisingly, getting the food after crying validates the message.

The quick reflexes that we develop when we sense heat are another good example of LTP. If you've burned your finger on a hot stove once or twice, then the third or fourth time your fingers get

close to the heat, you withdraw instinctively. You may even anticipate the pain of the burn. If you are subjected to certain painful
stimuli on a regular basis, then the perception of pain is just as
deeply imprinted as is the instinct to withdraw your hand from
the fire.

The Balance of Neurotransmitters

When a given set of neurons is stimulated in a repeated and predictable way, the response is reinforced and the circuitry becomes
hardwired. As we grow, the phenomenon of LTP remains an important function of the brain that enables us to learn more and more,
such as walking or playing a sport or an instrument. Such complex
tasks are best performed by second nature, in other words, through
a sophisticated yet subconscious neural network that developed as
a result of LTP. The two key neurotransmitters involved in LTP are
the amino acids glutamate and aspartate. Both are present in our
diets and are required for learning, and both are recycled as excitatory neurotransmitters in the postsynaptic neuron. While these
essential amino acids are required in ideal amounts for good health,
they have also been known to cause problems when present in high
amounts.

For example, excessive glutamate in the cerebrospinal fluid contributes to unhealthy excitatory responses, or central sensitivity. In
fact, the synthetic glutamate derivative **monosodium glutamate
(MSG)** has been associated with headaches and impaired learning
and is now prohibited in baby foods. Likewise, a derivative of
aspartate, N-methyl-D-aspartate (NMDA), facilitates learning and
the development of neural networks, but too much NMDA in the
central nervous system leads to a phenomenon called the "wind-up"
effect, which amplifies and perpetuates the pain message. For this
reason, a synthetic form of aspartate that is commercially available

---
Aspartame

Aspartame is the name for a noncarbohydrate sweetener, which is sold under a variety of trademark names. It can be found in about five thousand different foods and beverages, a large percentage of these being soft drinks and table condiments. It is unsuitable for baking because it breaks down chemically when exposed to heat. Some people have an intolerance to aspartame, and there have been studies investigating possible connections between aspartame and diseases such as brain tumors, brain lesions, and lymphoma, but nothing substantial has been discovered. The Food and Drug Administration has recognized some connections to symptoms such as abdominal pain, anxiety attacks, arthritis, asthma, bloating or edema, blood sugar control problems, some respiratory symptoms, an inability to concentrate, headaches, and other allergiclike reactions. Clearly, if you are experiencing these types of symptoms, it's worth cutting aspartame out of your diet to see whether you improve.

---

as a food sweetener (aspartame) has become a source of controversy due to its association with fibromyalgia symptoms. Removal of excitatory substances such as these from the diet has had a favorable effect on fibromyalgia in several studies.

Both glutamate and NMDA have been found in significantly higher levels in the cerebrospinal fluid of people who suffer from fibromyalgia, and the pain facilitators substance P and nerve growth factor have also been found at inappropriately high levels. These substances

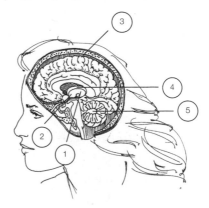

Key structures of the brain:
1—Thalamus, 2—Hypothalamus, 3—Sensory cortex, 4—Hippo-campus, 5—Cerebellum

are meant to exist in an optimal balance inside our brains and bodies—we need them to live healthy lives—but excessive amounts can make anyone miserable. Thus, in fibromyalgia, restoring neurotransmitters to their proper level of balance is pivotal to recovery.

With regard to the subtle imbalances of hormones and neurotransmitters in people with fibromyalgia, it isn't always clear whether the imbalance causes symptoms or is simply an innocent bystander. For example, impaired growth hormone responses have been observed in fibromyalgia sufferers, particularly in people who have fragmented sleep, but it is still unclear whether fibromyalgia symptoms actually arise because of this. Likewise, dopamine is a key inhibitory neurotransmitter that regulates muscle control, sleep, and pain perception, and low levels have been associated with central sensitivity. Since the absence of dopamine causes the tremors of Parkinson's disease, and excessive dopamine can cause psychosis, the importance of balance is clear. In fibromyalgia, a dampening of dopamine output from the nucleus accumbens is associated with stress-induced hyperalgesia. This finding has raised the idea of using a low dose of gentle **dopaminergic agents** to treat fibromyalgia. In fact, pramipexole (Mirapex), ordinarily used for **restless leg syndrome**, has shown early promise in alleviating fibromyalgia symptoms.

Unfortunately, the manipulation of only one neurotransmitter rarely provides meaningful long-term results. This is particularly true with fibromyalgia because central sensitivity tends to involve more than one neurotransmitter—not only dopamine, but serotonin, norepinephrine, gamma-aminobutyric acid (GABA), and others. This conundrum explains why the use of a **selective serotonin reuptake inhibitor (SSRI)** such as **fluoxetine** (Prozac) or **sertraline** (Zoloft) rarely provides any lasting relief for fibromyalgia sufferers. Or why **nonsteroidal anti-inflammatory drugs**

(NSAIDs) such as ibuprofen and naproxen are hardly ever effective for fibromyalgia because they inhibit only prostaglandin. For the same reason, narcotic analgesics such as morphine, codeine, and oxycodone, which are ideal for somatic pain due to their effect on opiate receptors, are largely inadequate in the treatment of fibromyalgia; they fail to address the many other causes of central imbalance. It is also one reason why this book offers a multi-pronged approach to treating fibromyalgia. With the multitude of symptoms, the involvement of different neurotransmitters, and the existence of widespread pain and discomfort, it's important to consider a variety of treatments: certain pharmaceuticals to address imbalances of neurotransmitters and provide pain relief, at least in the short term; and a whole host of nonpharmaceutical therapies such as supplements and vitamins, therapy, yoga, **tai chi**, and massage, chiropractic, and physical therapy. Don't put all of your hopes in one pill!

The results of clinical trials can sometimes make a new treatment appear better than it really is. For example, a new treatment for fibromyalgia may demonstrate a reduction of tender points by 25 percent, from twelve down to nine, and this might sound quite promising, but ask the woman who still has nine tender points whether she's satisfied and she may not be so enthusiastic. This healthy sense of skepticism is needed in fibromyalgia care because new treatments are studied every day, and the FDA reviews many of them.

Why do tender points develop in the first place? The answer is tricky since the root of the problem does not appear to be at the site of pain. When pain information arrives from the surface of the skin to the spinal cord, it crosses over to the opposite side of the spinal cord and travels up a pain pathway called the **spinothalamic tract** to the brain.

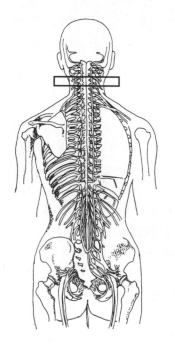
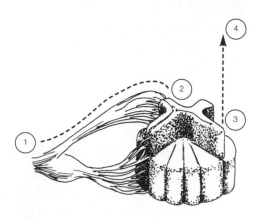

The pathways of pain: pain information arrives from the superficial tender points (1), travels to the posterior spinal cord (2), then crosses over to the opposite side of the cord (3), and ascends to the brain along the spinothalamic tract (4).

Inhibitory Neurotransmitters

When the messages of pain and other noxious stimuli arrive at the central nervous system, they are instantly down regulated by inhibitory neurotransmitters such as opiates, serotonin, GABA, and others; these are the counterparts to the excitatory messengers described earlier. They coexist in a proper balance among healthy individuals. Ultimately, the involved neurotransmitters—both inhibitory and excitatory—converge at the synapses of the spinal cord and the brain to determine the magnitude of the pain message. When this information is inappropriately amplified, we call this phenomenon central sensitivity, and this is the basic core of fibromyalgia, an imbalance that allows otherwise normal signals to be interpreted by the brain as painful or noxious.

Selected key structures in the brain involved in fibromyalgia are:

Thalamus, hypothalamus, HPA axis, and CRH center (the endocrine centers affected by stress regulate body weight, temperature, and many autonomic functions)

Sensory cortex (where sensation is ultimately perceived)

Hippocampus (where memory and behavior are affected)

Glial cells (the supporting architecture of neurons can propagate an inflammatory response inside the CNS)

Raphe nucleus (produces serotonin)

Locus ceruleus (produces norepinephrine)

Limbic system (**amygdala**, affects the CRH, the most primitive part of the CNS)

VLPO (ventrolateral preoptic) area (affects GABA and sleep)

Pain versus Suffering

Once the aberrant pain signal travels from the spinal cord to the thalamus, it is distributed to primitive and higher areas where the meaning of the pain must be interpreted. Pain signals arriving in the primitive limbic system create a sense of suffering or doom—a vague awareness that a threat exists—and this part of the brain may be abnormal on SPECT scanning in people with fibromyalgia. (SPECT scanning is single photon/positron emission computed tomography, or the injection of trace amounts of radio-labeled compounds that show up on a scan much as things do on an X-ray.)

It should be pointed out here that pain and suffering are not the same thing. Pain from a sprained ankle or a dental extraction has a perceived end point of recovery. You know that with each passing hour, you will feel better, until the pain has finally gone away.

Suffering, however, is the experience of pain—either physical or emotional—that doesn't seem to end, and from which you see no relief. Logically, this is associated with feelings of helplessness and hopelessness. In fibromyalgia, the boundaries of pain and suffering tend to merge.

In people who endure constant pain, it's hard to measure how much these individuals might be suffering. If people with fibromyalgia see the end in sight—a recovery, or the cessation of pain—they may be more likely to endure the discomfort. But if they endure day after day of backaches and muscle spasms, and they can't function, go to work, or enjoy their families, it's more than pain—it is pain and suffering. Physicians are better prepared to treat pain than suffering because suffering is not always something they can measure.

Betsy, a fibromyalgia sufferer, said that many clinicians tend not to address pain. Sometimes they dismiss the pain as psychiatric or become frustrated by their own inability to cure the patient. The physician needs to act with compassion, recognizing the pain and working to find a solution for it. With the fibromyalgia patient who suffers constantly, the physician needs to understand the important difference between pain and suffering, recognize both of them as real, and do his or her best to treat the whole person.

The physician who is a whiz clinician may not understand how the pain impacts the patient, and our current medical system doesn't always allow the physician

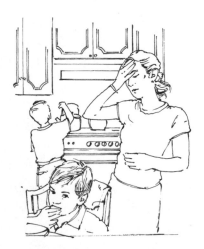

Feelings of suffering and despair can be overwhelming in people with fibromyalgia.

to spend more than ten minutes discussing how the pain affects the patient's life. In some cases, a sense of purpose and a strong work ethic help people to work through the pain and avoid some of the suffering, but if it is misery without meaning and without the empathy of caregivers, then the pain merges into the realm of suffering. Suffering also contributes to chronic stress, which, as we have seen, harms the person in the long term. Suffering is fundamentally an emotional condition, but it is as real as pain and must be taken into account whenever a physician evaluates someone.

The Higher Centers of Pain Reception

From the thalamus, the pain message is sent to the hypothalamus (which regulates endocrine function), the hippocampus (memory), the frontal cortex (behavior), and the sensory cortex (which determines the specific location of pain). What is most fascinating is that central sensitivity creates an environment of sensitivity in the generally pain-free regions of the body (the bulky muscles), while the most sensitive parts (eye, tongue, genitals, etc.) are rarely affected by fibromyalgia. In addition, fibromyalgia is only one part of the spectrum of central sensitivity, which also includes migraine headache; irritable bowel; insomnia; sensitivity to chemicals, bright lights, and loud noises; and possibly allergic responses and autoimmune illnesses. Each of these phenomena can be exacerbated by stress, particularly in susceptible individuals.

In such cases, the primitive stress response that protects us from danger can become overtaxed. Exposure to mild stress or occasional stress is unavoidable, and our nervous systems are equipped to deal with this, but an unhealthy atmosphere of constant stress and tension causes a dysregulation of the stress-response system

---
The Stress-Response System

We've all experienced moments of stress, ranging from car accidents to sudden unemployment or the deaths of loved ones, and most of us have the skills to deal with events like these. During an emergency, we have a fight-or-flight response that gets the adrenaline pumping and gives us extra energy until we return to our normal state.

Now, imagine a child in an abusive home who lives in constant fear, listening to his or her parents argue and throw things around. Eventually, the child remains in a continual state of readiness and carries this hypervigilance into adulthood. Remember long-term potentiation—the child learns that certain behaviors in the mother will result in other behaviors in the father. The child is unable to control either parent, but he or she may unconsciously react to certain situations. Later, when the child becomes a teen or a young adult, a shouting man, no matter how benign the situation, may create the same stress response. The constant overproduction of cortisol, the anxiety of feeling unsafe, hard-wires this young person to be hyper-alert. When we consider the sensitivity of the stress-response system, it's easy to understand why someone like this may be more likely to have fibromyalgia in adulthood.

Post-Traumatic Stress Disorder

Post-traumatic stress disorder, which gained widespread recognition after veterans returned from the Vietnam and the Gulf wars with symptoms, affects many people besides veterans. Imagine what 9/11 was like for people who survived the attack on the World Trade Center towers. Low-flying planes, sirens, or screams would bring them right back to that moment. It doesn't have to be war or a terrorist attack, either. Other common causes of PTSD are rape, sexual assault, childhood abuse, or a physical attack. Today we know that some people carry the impact of such abuse for years afterward and eventually become prone to developing fibromyalgia. Their humiliating memories interfere with a sense of security and contribute to fragmented sleep. Not surprisingly, a person with fibromyalgia develops a feeling that he or she lacks control over the bad things that happen in life. It isn't that every fibromyalgia sufferer has PTSD, but when it exists, whether acknowledged or not, it can predispose the person to develop fibromyalgia later in life. Remember, again, the impact of stress hormones on the hippocampus, and how the brain becomes physically changed. The person also goes through life feeling somewhat threatened and perhaps without the positive outlook that another individual may take for granted.

With PTSD and the development of fibromyalgia, adverse early life events typically get the ball rolling. A single traumatic episode or an environment of constant fear or insecurity causes hypervigilance and hyperactivity of the stress response system. This, in turn, leads to maladaptive pain behavior and susceptibility to fibromyalgia. The increased sensitivity resulting from chronic stress causes muscle, facial, and ocular tension; hyperawareness; headaches; insomnia; and painful trigger points. Perhaps this is why posttraumatic stress frequently manifests with physical symptoms, and why people with fibromyalgia have a threefold increase of reported post-traumatic stress compared to other painful conditions. In fact, childhood abuse has been associated with measurable changes within the hippocampus, although the development of fibromyalgia in such susceptible individuals often requires a second stressor later in life.

Stress, Memory, and "Fibro-Fog"

In response to chronic stress, measurable changes have been found in the corticotropin-releasing hormone center and the **locus ceruleus-norepinephrine** center, which ultimately affect their

---

"Fibro-Fog"

A teacher diagnosed with fibromyalgia took a leave of absence because "fibro-fog" made it impossible for her to remember what to do when she got into the classroom. She showed up, then forgot all of her normal cues. A trial lawyer, after suffering a series of stressful incidents in childhood, was in a car accident as an adult and then suddenly couldn't recall important details in the courtroom.

Problems with memory, or fibro-fog, are worse than forgetting where you put your keys or failing to pick up the dry cleaning. Imagine going in to do the job you've done for ten years and suddenly not remembering anything—this is the curse of fibro-fog.

---

downstream targets: the HPA axis (regulating cortisone) and the sympathetic nervous system (regulating adrenaline). The resulting imbalance of the stress-response system leads to neuronal damage and atrophy of several vulnerable structures. Damage to the sensitive hippocampus (where memories are processed and stored) is associated with poor concentration and the "fibro-fog" so commonly described by sufferers.

The short-term memory, or working memory, stores most of the day-to-day details. The rest goes into the long-term memory. When we fail to remember something, we tend to think our ability to retrieve the information is lacking. What might really be happening is that we are concentrating less and thus remembering less and failing to multitask. Fortunately, the kind of memory problems that fibromyalgia sufferers have tends to be with focus or attention, which usually can improve with practice.

If you would like to boost your mental skills, tell yourself that your memory is good. Your mind will then try to prove that this is true; it's a matter of positive thinking. Another technique that develops your memory is simply to pay better attention to things. It helps if a topic is interesting and important to you because then you do this naturally, but if you make the effort, you'll see results. Relating new material to something you already know will help. Also, try explaining what you have learned to someone else. This helps to imprint the details in your own mind. Organize your notes so that you can review them later. And use all your senses. Some of us are better at reading new material and remembering it; others need to see it. Visualize information to help you retain it, and use mnemonics, devising words or sentences out of facts, then creating a mental picture to help you remember it. For instance, to remember something about George Washington, think of young George with an ax and a chopped-down cherry tree.

We all deal with some level of confusion or memory loss, but for various reasons people with fibromyalgia may experience this in more intense ways. For one thing, intense pain and discomfort may make it difficult for them to concentrate on things the way they'd like to. The sensations of pain and fatigue crowd out anything else they need to focus on. Depression and sleep deprivation have the same effect on memory and concentration. For example, a car accident that results from an inability to concentrate triggers even more sleeplessness and anxiety. If you don't sleep well, as many fibromyalgia sufferers don't, then it's difficult to pay attention to all the details of daily living. There is a direct connection between sleep and the production of serotonin (which aids memory). Decreased blood flow to certain areas of the brain may also lead to problems with short-term memory. Chronic pain actually inhibits the brain's ability to create memories. The processing of pain signals takes up a lot of the brain's time and energy and reduces the amount of time spent creating new memories. This, coupled with stress, leaves us without the resources to remember some of the simple things in life.

It might not be as severe as having a car accident because you can't focus, but certainly losing your keys, driving away with your coffee mug on top of your car, leaving your purse in the grocery store shopping basket, or forgetting medications are all things that can happen as a result of fibro-fog.

Try to maintain a healthy sleeping environment; allow your doctor to treat you for depression or sleep deprivation because these things will only snowball into other areas of your life. Stay busy by doing things that keep your mind active. Read, do crosswords or jigsaws, or see a play. This will require a little physical exertion on your part, but it might help you to cut through the layers of fibro-fog. Physical exercise, in moderation, also helps you to be more alert.

Don't be embarrassed by occasional lapses in memory. It doesn't happen only to people with fibromyalgia or individuals who are developing dementia or Alzheimer's disease. Everybody forgets things. Everybody does something silly now and then. Explain to your family and close friends what is going on. Perhaps your spouse can do a quick check before you walk out in the morning—do you have your keys, your lunch, your purse, your cell phone? Don't let this make you feel like a child; allow people to help you. Besides, the more your family and close friends support you in this, the better you will feel.

Avoid distractions. If your teenager insists on playing loud music next to the kitchen where you are trying to do some paperwork, get him or her some headphones. Move away from the TV, loud conversations, or other background noise, which only make your attempt to concentrate more of a struggle.

The foregoing advice may make fibro-fog seem like a mere inconvenience, requiring only minimal efforts to fix things. Yet this isn't always the case. As we mentioned earlier, the teacher who went into her classroom and couldn't remember what to do next was suffering from more extreme symptoms. Fibro-fog can be a minor hassle, or it can be an impairment that affects the very essence of your life. Obviously, fibro-fog can be one of the most upsetting and troubling symptoms of fibromyalgia.

Symptoms of Fibro-Fog

- Short-term memory loss
- Trouble remembering where you put things
- Trouble remembering plans
- Difficulty retaining new information
- A tendency to transpose letters and numbers
- Trouble concentrating and focusing
- Trouble remembering simple numbers (like PIN numbers for bank cards!)
- Problems with language, including difficulty holding conversations, understanding what others are saying, and expressing thoughts
- Problems finding just the right words to use in a conversation

---

People may experience memory loss, difficulties using language, and problems with learning. They might feel as if they are in a haze or a fog, hence the name "fibro-fog." This mental state can occur at any time, triggered by stress, anxiety, pain, or seemingly by nothing at all. Pain seems to intensify these symptoms.

Perhaps the fibro-fog will last only a few days, or maybe it will cloud your mind for weeks or months. If you recognize it as one more symptom of the overall condition known as fibromyalgia, discuss it with your physician and family, and treat it appropriately, the effects can be minimized. Otherwise, fibro-fog just adds more stress to an otherwise difficult period of your life.

Inflammation and Chronic Stress

Is there an inflammatory component to all of this? Strangely enough, the answer is yes. A mild inflammatory response is actually driven by chronic stress. Though imperceptible by standard blood tests, elevated levels of various circulating **cytokines** (inflammatory mediators) such as tumor necrosis factor (**TNF-alpha**) and **interleukin-1** have been identified. These cytokines contribute to the flulike aching and fatigue of fibromyalgia and can amplify the pain message as well. The cells in the central nervous system most likely responsible for producing cytokines are the glial cells, which are derived from immune cell lineage. Glial cells are not involved in normal everyday pain perception, but they become activated during pathological situations, such as chronic illness or in the setting of a stubborn pain generator. In this way, the immune system and the brain have a powerful connection, and this might explain how emotional triggers can exacerbate certain immunological disorders such as systemic lupus, multiple sclerosis, psoriasis, and Crohn's disease.

Is there anything you can do about inflammation? Possibly, there is. Many nutrition books have been published recently on the benefits of an anti-inflammation diet to alleviate autoimmune disease symptoms, help to prevent heart disease and cancer, and foster a state of optimal health. It isn't within the scope of this book to describe the anti-inflammation diet, but the literature is available for people who want to take control of their health.

The Psychosomatic Link

That is not to say that stress causes any of the conditions listed previously, but there is an undeniable link involved, a psychosomatic link that should not be dismissed. There are emotional-mental aspects, as well as physical, in every part of our lives. For instance, after a particularly stressful event, like the death of a loved one, a person may stop eating or sleeping normally for some time. These are real physical manifestations of an emotional event.

Naturally, both skepticism and concern arise at the notion of psychosomatic illness, so let's be clear: the pain of fibromyalgia is real. The suffering is real, and there are very real objective changes in the brains of people with fibromyalgia. Yet let us not deny the physical manifestations of central sensitivity that are, by strict definition, psychosomatic. People who are most open-minded about this concept are always the first to recover.

3

Pain Generators

You would think that a person with chronic pain would eventually get used to it, but, unfortunately, the opposite is true. Untreated, chronic pain leads only to more pain. In fact, any source of chronic pain, even a minor one, can activate the body's central pain pathways and sensitize the brain in a very detrimental way. This occurs in part because the neurotransmitters of pain—substance P, glutamate, NMDA receptors, nerve growth factors, and inflammatory cytokines (such as TNF-alpha)—circulate in greater amounts inside the cerebrospinal fluid and cause the brain to interpret more pain than actually exists.

In the world of fibromyalgia, a stubborn, unyielding source of chronic pain is known as a pain generator. Whenever a pain generator exists in the body, a faster and more efficient transmission of the pain message ultimately occurs, the body's fields of pain are expanded, and the central receptors for pain are sensitized. Not only do you anticipate the pain, but the body actually sends the message more quickly and intensely, making the pain impossible to ignore. To make matters worse, the fibromyalgia itself becomes its own source of chronic pain, yet another feedback loop to further perpetuate the problem of central sensitivity!

Temporary, acute pain is not the issue here. A bad sunburn or the pain of an ankle sprain does not last long enough to cause central sensitivity. A failed back operation, however, or a difficult labor and delivery can produce symptoms of pain, impairment, and despair that stick around just long enough to sensitize the central pathways of pain. Pain generators, as far as fibromyalgia is concerned, must activate the central pathways long enough to affect changes in pain processing due to a constant pain message, not just a fleeting one. For example, the neuropathic pain that sometimes persists after a bad case of shingles or the relentless pain of a herniated cervical disk can lead to lasting changes in pain transmission.

Consider Nancy, a thirty-five-year-old mother of two, who has suffered from lower-back pain for several years. Although she is upbeat and active, after months of living with constant pain, she developed the symptoms of fibromyalgia. **Positive thinking**, yoga, and analgesics can't stop her from being aware of the pain every morning when she wakes up. Not only that, she anticipates the sensation of pain and finds herself guarding every movement as if it might exacerbate this pain. What started as a backache and was left untreated ultimately changed the way her body reacted to painful stimuli. Now she understands the necessity of resolving the back pain in order to control all the other symptoms.

In Nancy's case, a lumbar spine MRI scan revealed an extruded disk fragment that had been pressing on one of her spinal nerve roots. She needed surgery, which was highly successful and led to her ultimate recovery.

A pain generator isn't always this elusive, but it is always relevant. The amplification of pain is a correctable mistake—a misguided message—that occurs every day inside the brains of people with fibromyalgia. For this reason, the complete recovery from fibromyalgia requires a thoughtful search for, and the eradication of, all pain generators. Once this is accomplished, the vicious cycle can be broken.

Finding the Responsible Pain Generators

A pain generator can be **mechanical** or **nonmechanical**. Most mechanical pain generators arise after trauma, although some are developmental, postural, or degenerative in nature. A few examples of mechanical pain generators are whiplash, myofascial pain, and chronic back pain.

In susceptible people, a nonmechanical pain generator can also lead to nonrestorative sleep, a poor sense of well-being, and a source of chronic discomfort that drives the fibromyalgia process. Examples of nonmechanical pain generators are the joint pains of systemic lupus or Lyme disease, the muscle aching of thyroid dysregulation, and the burning nerve pain of peripheral neuropathy.

When Pain and Depression Converge

In some cases, mechanical and nonmechanical sources of pain occur together and overwhelm the central pathways. An example of this is a person with chronic depression who suffers a slip-and-fall injury, followed by a progression to fibromyalgia. This unfortunate confluence of events activates the central pathways inherently shared by sensation and emotion, escalating both problems. For this reason, dual inhibitors of both serotonin and norepinephrine are being used to treat the problems of depression and chronic pain that commonly occur in the same person.

Many people with fibromyalgia declare, "You'd be depressed, too, if you had all of this pain. You'd be stressed, too, if you were in constant discomfort." These complaints sound reasonable, but their causes and effects are not so simple. Many people with painful arthritic conditions are not the least bit depressed, and just as many depressed people have no pain at all. It's the convergence of the two—the umbrella of fibromyalgia under which pain and despair coexist—that demands our attention. The common central pathways of sensation are both tactile and emotional, and it is here that the answers will be found.

Unlike Nancy, who suffered pain because of an extruded disk fragment, Christine, a few years older and employed as an executive secretary, experienced the onset of fibromyalgia in her midthirties. Without any warning, she found that her moods were dark. She felt hopeless about the future, was often tired during the day, and was unable to function at her usual pace. Although she was diagnosed with fibromyalgia soon after the onset of symptoms, finding the right balance of pharmaceuticals was a challenge. The pervasive feelings of depression affected her as much as the fatigue and the pain did. In addition, the fatigue, pain, and depression were so intertwined that treatment had to address all three aspects simultaneously. Her physician was able to ease Nancy's depression with a low dose of a common antidepressant. As her mood lifted, she became better able to cope with the pain of fibromyalgia. Analgesics, when appropriate, eased her discomfort, and she began a well-thought-out course of recovery that combined emotional support, yoga, an appropriate diet, and nutritional supplements. It wasn't one specific medication or therapy but the combination of remedies that enabled her to look beyond the hopelessness, feel positive, and begin to feel better overall.

Selected Mechanical and
——————————— Nonmechanical Pain Generators ———————————

The seven types of mechanical pain generators that can perpetuate fibromyalgia are:

1. Whiplash

2. Chronic lower-back pain, including herniated disks, degenerative disk disease (neck or back), scoliosis, and spondylosis (osteoarthritis of the spine)

3. Arnold-Chiari malformation and other forms of posterior cervical spinal cord compression

4. Myofascial pain, especially around the neck or the lower back (this includes thoracic outlet syndrome and the muscle tension that can arise from a pelvic obliquity or a leg-length discrepancy)

5. TMJ and other facial pain syndromes, chronic headache, and trigeminal neuralgia

6. Arthritis, tendonitis, and bursitis, especially around the neck, the shoulder, or the hip

7. Unhealed injuries, fracture pain, phantom pain, **reflex sympathetic dystrophy (RSD)**, and postincision pain

The seven types of nonmechanical pain generators that can perpetuate fibromyalgia are:

1. Neuropathic: diabetic neuropathy, frostbite injury, multiple sclerosis, burn injuries, postherpetic neuralgia, and peripheral vascular infarction

2. Rheumatological conditions: systemic lupus, postvasculitis, rheumatoid arthritis, myositis, polymyalgia rheumatica, and ankylosing spondylitis

3. Encephalopathy: postconcussion, traumatic brain injury, ischemic (poststroke), depression, and bipolar disorder

4. Postinfectious: Lyme disease, hepatitis C, HIV, Epstein-Barr virus, and others

5. Drug side effects: lipid-lowering agents (statins), protease inhibitors (for HIV), bisphosphonates (for osteoporosis), and rarely SSRIs (for depression).

6. Endocrine syndromes: thyroid disorders, parathyroid and adrenal disorders, acromegaly, and hemochromatosis

7. Cancer (rare): including paraneoplastic disease, metastatic disease, pancreatic cancer, and renal cell carcinoma

---

Whiplash as a Pain Generator

With regard to fibromyalgia, the most pernicious pain generator is probably whiplash. How often do you hear of someone being rear ended in an accident? It happens all the time; many of us have experienced whiplash. Only recently, though, have physicians (and not all physicians) made the connection between whiplash and the subsequent development of fibromyalgia. The fact that you can have a whiplash injury long before you develop fibromyalgia makes it even harder for patients and their physicians to figure out cause and effect.

This type of injury leads to fibromyalgia in up to 20 percent of motor vehicle accident victims, particularly in susceptible individuals. It occurs for several reasons, some of which include a silent and unforeseen injury to the brain and the cervical spinal cord, a tendency of the injury to remain as a chronic source of neck pain, and the emotional impact often associated with a car accident (anxiety, insomnia, anger, fear, time off work, etc.).

Common problems arise after whiplash because its victims don't take the injuries seriously enough and don't treat them quickly enough. Remarkably, this is also true among doctors in the urgent-care setting who are satisfied when X-rays do not show fractures, and they send patients home with little more than prescriptions for rest and a brief course of pain medicine. The truth is that whiplash needs to be treated promptly in a multifaceted way with manual therapy (such as chiropractic), muscle relaxants, and passive stretching *before* the muscle tension sets in.

On the surface, a person who has suffered whiplash will complain of escalating neck pain, muscular stiffness, regional tingling, and sometimes chest pain, nausea, or dizziness. The actual injury runs deeper, however, and few doctors are able to recognize it. If you ask ten doctors what happens to the head and the neck after whiplash, you will probably get ten different answers. In reality, whiplash causes at least three types of injury:

1. The first injury is entirely mechanical, a ligament injury that results from the violent hyperextension and hyperflexion of the cervical spine. Recall that the ligaments are the tensile structures that connect bone to bone (or one vertebra to the next), and they do not heal rapidly. Damaged ligaments can take months to heal, and very few available treatments can successfully speed up the process. In some cases, the force of a car accident results in a hidden bone contusion, a spinal cord injury, or a hairline fracture in one of the cervical vertebrae, all potential sources of chronic pain.

2. Several days to weeks after the initial whiplash event, myofascial pain sets in. At first, the muscle spasm that develops after a neck injury serves to protect the spinal cord, not unlike a natural cervical collar. Yet the persistence of spasm leads to a painful shortening of muscle fibers and the development of trigger points or knots within the paracervical muscle groups, also known as myofascial triggers. Left alone, myofascial pain usually gets worse. In fact, there's no good pill for this problem, which underscores its prevalence, since pharmaceuticals have been such a mainstay of treatment in modern medicine. Ultimately, this common sequel of whiplash requires a hands-on approach such

as myofascial release therapy, chiropractic, or physical therapy for a successful outcome.

3. Finally, the most insidious injury caused by whiplash is the silent brain injury, one that can persist for months or years after the original accident. While the problem might not be immediately apparent, the results of a silent brain injury, usually starting as a concussion (from the sensitive brain rattling around inside a hard, closed skull) can be most vexing to identify and treat. Although any part of the brain or the spinal cord can be affected, the sensitive hippocampus and the superficial sensory cortex are most exposed to injury and contribute, in no small part, to the postwhiplash fibromyalgia so commonly seen. The hippocampus, where memory is stored, is particularly vulnerable, which explains the impairment of cognitive function, a common symptom of fibromyalgia.

It suffices to say that in the emergency room setting or the doctor's office, whiplash is approached (with the best of intentions)

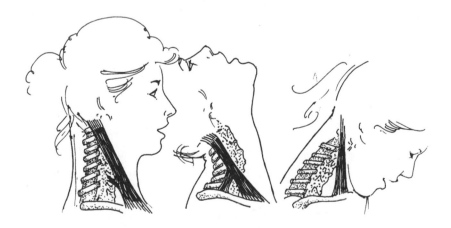

Whiplash causes a ligamentous injury, followed soon afterward by a myofascial pain syndrome. In some cases, whiplash is associated with a postconcussion brain injury and may be a source of post traumatic stress.

What Happens in Whiplash

An adult head weighs about eight pounds, or as much as a bowling ball, and in a sudden stop, when the head is thrown forward violently, this puts a brief but extreme strain on the neck. The immediate reflex contraction completes the injury. Headache, dizziness, and abnormal sensations such as burning or pricking, shoulder or back pain, and concentration or memory problems are all common. Because X-rays don't show damage to soft tissue, a CT scan or an MRI may be necessary to get a more detailed look at injuries. Treatment for whiplash remains quite basic, although the extent of this injury can require much more aggressive treatment.

---

with a plain cervical spine X-ray, NSAIDs, muscle relaxants, and analgesics, and quite often patients will recover without any untoward complications. If there is no evidence of fracture and the patient is medically stable, the whiplash victim may be uneventfully discharged from the acute-care setting, although he or she is best advised to visit a chiropractor or an osteopath within a few days after the accident in order to begin some gentle mobilization.

Reactive Fibromyalgia

Strangely enough, while seat belts have saved lives in recent years, they have probably contributed to a higher rate of whiplash injuries. In addition, **reactive fibromyalgia**—the fibromyalgia that occurs after a sudden physical trauma—is often more stubborn and difficult to treat than are other types, and it typically lasts for years. For this reason, a whiplash ligament injury (including the consequences of myofascial pain and silent brain injury), which can eventually become a hardwired vehicle for fibromyalgia and central sensitivity, should always be taken seriously and treated promptly.

The Question of Inflammation after Trauma

Can an injury cause inflammation? Certainly, it can. If you suffer an ankle sprain or a fractured finger, there is obvious swelling, warmth, and redness immediately afterward. This is an example of the body's immune system sending the necessary messengers of repair to the site of the injury—an attempt to get rid of the injured debris in order to begin the process of repair.

An inflammatory response may be okay for skin and bone, which can easily replicate and function well in the setting of a scar, but the nervous system is most unforgiving when it comes to such matters. A nervous system injury—a stroke, a severed nerve, encephalitis, or oxygen deprivation—is invariably followed by a deficit. Brain matter, the spinal cord, and the peripheral nerves do not regenerate the way other organ systems do. The body does not have nerve tissue in abundance the way it has excess kidney or lung or liver cells. For this reason, researchers believe that shutting down the body's inflammatory response immediately after a CNS injury might lead to less damage in the long run. This is already being demonstrated in the area of stroke and head injury, and there are similar implications as far as fibromyalgia is concerned. The earliest interventions always make the greatest difference in the long run. Studies using **interleukin-10**, a naturally occurring anti-inflammatory cytokine, are underway.

Other Pain Generators

There is an association between headaches and pain near the temporomandibular joint (TMJ), or jawbone, in people who have fibromyalgia. It makes sense that if these sources of pain exist in conjunction with fibromyalgia, the physician and the patient need to take a good long look at why this is happening. Stress might contribute to either a headache or TMJ, but ruling out other physical causes of this pain and reducing the pain as much as possible can only benefit the fibromyalgia sufferer.

Headache

Up to 50 percent of people with fibromyalgia complain of chronic headaches, and most of these are typical migraines. This suggests a common etiology between the two conditions. In some cases, the link between fibromyalgia and headache may be seen in people who get tension headaches, arising from daily stress or referred pain due to a myofascial trigger point. Sometimes, the muscular sources of head and neck pain can actually trigger a migraine. Thus, a better understanding of headache and its causes can benefit the person who has fibromyalgia.

Migraine headaches have long been thought to arise from the dilation of blood vessels inside the head, resulting in the compression of other areas. Thus, the treatments for migraines have been proposed accordingly—such as, give a vasoconstrictor for relief—and in many cases, this remedy has worked well for people with migraines. Yet the concept of vascular dilation and constriction is probably too simplistic and inadequate to explain the many other aspects of migraine. The prodrome of food cravings, yawning, and concurrent mood changes so commonly described with migraines implicate an imbalance of dopamine inside the central nervous system. The well-described nausea and the aura of strange smells and altered lights further suggest a central imbalance, or central sensitization.

In all likelihood, the excitability inside the brain is reflective of some of the same sources—the overabundance of excitatory amino acids, substance P dysregulation, and psychosomatic triggers that exacerbate both migraine headaches and fibromyalgia. In addition, some of the demographics—a preponderance of women, a history of stressful events or head injury, obesity, and documented sleep disturbances—are also strangely similar between the two conditions.

Treating a migraine, separate from all the issues of fibromyalgia, can include preventive care, using medications and/or supplements like magnesium and vitamin B6; avoiding triggers (not necessarily stress) such as changes in the weather and air pressure, certain foods, aspartame, and MSG; using cerebral vasoconstrictor abortive agents; and undertaking effective pain management.

For more information on migraine and tension headaches, please see pages 135–136 in chapter 9.

TMJ Syndrome

Nearly 75 percent of people who have fibromyalgia will complain of pain near the temporomandibular joint, or jawbone, at some point in their lives. This is a staggering figure, but it's not surprising when you consider the mechanics involved. Some orthodontists still attribute the TMJ syndrome to a **malocclusion** of the bite, and while this may be true on occasion, there's little reason to suspect this in most cases. The truth is that 90 percent of TMJ is

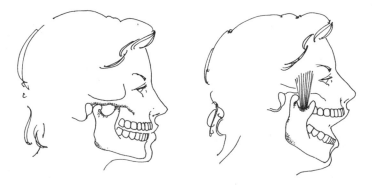

Temporomandibular joint pain is usually driven by myofascial pain of the temporalis and buccinator muscles. Teeth grinding at night (bruxism) and chronic stress may contribute to this.

related to the surrounding muscles of mastication—the **masseter**, the **buccinator**, and the **temporalis**—muscles that are prone to myofascial pain and shortening. During periods of stress, these powerful muscles easily overwhelm the relatively small TMJ and its disk, and this leads to the disturbing sensations of clicking, crunching, and chronic pain.

The problem of TMJ typically begins at night during the early stages of sleep when one experiences the phenomenon of teeth grinding—also known as **bruxism**—a manifestation of daytime stress. Consequently, the pain in and around the TMJ leads to additional tension or myofascial pain of the facial muscles, and TMJ syndrome becomes a responsible pain generator. A vicious cycle ultimately sets in when TMJ syndrome, combined with emotional stress, insomnia, and pain amplification, all feed off one another to perpetuate the greater problem of fibromyalgia.

A common treatment approach to TMJ, largely advocated by members of the dental profession, is a bite plate designed to protect the teeth from grinding and to realign a perceived malocclusion. The more contemporary and successful approaches, however, include relaxation of the involved muscles via massage, myofascial release, transcranial magnetic stimulation (rTMS), ultrasound, and (when necessary) a temporary prescription for a muscle relaxant (usually in the Valium family). Surgical treatment for TMJ can be successful, but it is best to explore all the nonsurgical options first. Ultimately, greater insight into stress reduction makes sense for people who suffer from both TMJ and fibromyalgia syndrome.

Arnold-Chiari Malformation

Arnold-Chiari malformation is an anatomical defect where the lower brain meets the upper cervical spinal canal. It is defined as a herniation, or a "squeezing through," of the lowest part of the brain—the **cerebellar tonsils**—to at least 3 to 5 mm below the

foramen magnum (the canal through which the spinal cord descends). This has neurological implications that include headaches, numbness, clumsiness, and issues regarding incontinence, and it has been discovered in recent years that the discomfort and the fatigue associated with a type 1 Chiari malformation are strikingly similar to fibromyalgia. Although this is still a somewhat controversial area, enough people with fibromyalgia have been found to have an associated Chiari malformation that routine screening or at least a healthy suspicion is advisable. The diagnosis can be made by an MRI scan of the upper cervical spine, and anyone who is found to have a Chiari malformation may benefit from surgery.

─────── **A Surgical Remedy for Chiari Malformation** ───────

Although the incidence of Arnold-Chiari malformation in fibromyalgia is only 0.5 percent (or 1 in 200), the outcome for corrective surgery for Arnold-Chiari is usually good, with most patients seeing real improvement in their symptoms. Sometimes the symptoms of Chiari malformation may be unmasked by a car accident or another trauma; the underlying condition is congenital. The surgery requires a recuperation of about two months—sometimes more—and repeated trauma can bring on a recurrence of symptoms.

Neuropathic Pain

Neuropathic pain, as the name implies, is a pathological source of pain that arises from within the nervous system itself, usually due to damage at the level of the peripheral nerves that is most often caused by diabetes, peripheral vascular disease, chemotherapy, or herpes zoster (shingles). This damage causes an exaggerated response to external noxious stimuli, an expansion of peripheral pain fields, and a persistence of the pain message instead of the normal winding down. Normally, if you stub your toe, there is a crescendo of pain that comes to a peak within a few seconds, after which the pain quickly subsides. This is an example of central inhibition coming to the rescue. Yet people who have neuropathic pain lack this protective mechanism, and fibromyalgia syndrome is within the spectrum of this problem.

The quality of neuropathic pain is somewhat different from the throbbing ache of arthritis or the sharp pain of an ear infection. Neuropathy causes more of an obnoxious burning and tingling sensation, typically in an extremity or around the torso due to the involvement of a peripheral nerve. Sometimes neuropathic pain is central in origin, such as the pain that is sometimes seen after a stroke or in people with multiple sclerosis. Certain individuals experience fibromyalgia syndrome after recovering from encephalitis—the brain infection that can occur from chicken pox, Lyme disease, Epstein-Barr virus, and so many other infections.

Most doctors think of the term *neuropathy* as peripheral neuropathy, which implies an injury to, or a dysfunction of, the peripheral nerves between the spinal cord and the skin due to diabetes or poor circulation. There are so many different kinds of neuropathy, and just as many causes, including postzoster (shingles) neuropathy, frostbite injury, chemotherapy, vasculitis (inflammation of the blood vessels), **amyloidosis** (the accumulation of an insoluble protein fiber around the nerves), heavy metal toxicity, and others. The diagnosis can be made by a physician taking a good history and conducting a physical exam, and a neurologist or a physiatrist giving the patient an electromyelogram.

In addition to disorders of the peripheral nerves, the central nervous system should also be included in this category, since the centralization of pain is, by definition, neuropathic. The features of fibromyalgia known as **allodynea** (the misinterpretation of normal touch as pain) and **hyperalgesia** (abnormally high sensitivity to pain) are, in all likelihood, centrally driven. In either case, any painful neuropathy can serve as a responsible pain generator in susceptible patients, not only by amplifying the constant pain of fibromyalgia but also by feeding the process of central sensitivity. In fact, it is very common for people with fibromyalgia to complain of subjective tingling or burning of the extremities, even in the setting of a normal electromyelogram.

NEUROPATHIC DAMAGE

- Damage to peripheral nerves
- Ectopic discharge
- Recruitment of noninjured nerve fibers
- Loss of central inhibition
- Development of central sensitization

Interestingly, the mechanisms of neuropathic pain share several features with fibromyalgia. These may include the loss of central inhibition (the brain's failure to produce soothing endorphins in response to a noxious stimulus) and the recruitment of noninjured nerve fibers into the pain message (resulting in an ordinarily innocuous sensation being interpreted as noxious). Both fibromyalgia and peripheral neuropathy also share favorable responses to certain agents, such as **alpha-2 delta receptor blockers** and agents designed to correct the central imbalance of serotonin and norepinephrine. Perhaps of greatest importance, both conditions arise from damage to the nervous system and respond best to a combination of treatments rather than to a single drug.

Reflex Sympathetic Dystrophy

Reflex sympathetic dystrophy (RSD), also known as **complex regional pain syndrome**, is a disorder that typically affects one extremity at a time but can also affect more than one. The constant and noxious pain of RSD fits best within the spectrum of neuropathic pain, although the level of injury is probably at the spinal cord instead of at a peripheral nerve. There is also a vascular quality to the problem of RSD that contributes to swelling of an extremity, temperature or color changes, hypersensitivity to touch, excessive sweating, and eventual atrophy of the underlying bone and muscle.

The three stages of reflex sympathetic dystrophy are:

1. Pain in a limb that usually, but not always, follows an injury. The injury is frequently proximal to the pain; for example, a shoulder or neck injury may be followed by painful swelling of a hand. Notwithstanding injury, painful RSD can emerge after a stroke, a heart attack, or surgery such as an arthroscopy. The pain is usually burning or throbbing, with localized edema and sensitivity to touch.

2. There is progression of soft tissue swelling during stage 2, with escalation of sensitivity and pain that can last up to six months. For the best chance of a complete recovery, it is crucial to intervene prior to the late development of this stage.

3. The swelling begins to subside in this late stage, replaced by atrophy of the surrounding muscle and contracture of the underlying tissues (such as the hand or the fingers). Although there is no further visible swelling, the pain is just as severe and it persists.

In the majority of cases of RSD, an injury immediately precedes its development, and quite often a significant emotional disturbance occurs at the same time. Doctors have long recognized the painful swelling that can strangely affect a hand after a more proximal shoulder injury—originally known as shoulder-hand syndrome—and still, there's no clear explanation of why this happens. The growing consensus among pain specialists is that the persistent injury at the level of the spinal cord, and the ongoing damage to its tributaries—the peripheral nerves—might actually be inflammatory in nature. This theory has opened the door to new treatment possibilities by addressing the immune system effects, as well as the pain itself.

The diagnosis of RSD can be made by an astute clinician, aided by certain imaging techniques such as bone scanning, X-rays, and MRI scanning. The real trick is to identify RSD as early as possible before it advances to a late stage.

Rheumatological and Inflammatory Sources of Pain

There are more than a hundred different kinds of arthritis, any of which can serve as a source of chronic pain. The one that's most prevalent in the population is osteoarthritis (OA), the wear-and-tear deterioration of cartilage that is most troubling to the fibromyalgia sufferer when it affects the cervical spine. This is also known as **cervical spondylosis**, which includes degenerative disk disease, vertebral spurs, and facet joint arthritis (wear and tear of the facet joints that ordinarily enable fluid rotation of the neck). In some cases, the responsible pain generator will be OA elsewhere, such as the lower back, shoulder, hip, or knee, any of which can interrupt sleep and amplify central pain.

When there is overlapping OA, options for treatment are myriad, and these will be discussed in part II. It suffices to say that the proper treatment of painful OA in people with fibromyalgia can have immeasurably beneficial effects. There are also many inflammatory types of arthritis, the most common of which is rheumatoid arthritis (RA), although RA is not as strongly associated with fibromyalgia as one might imagine. When the two conditions coexist, the proper treatment of RA, which includes a highly effective assortment of biological agents these days, can dramatically reduce the associated fibromyalgia complaints.

Sometimes overlooked as a source of inflammatory arthritis is a condition that affects the lower back and the sacroiliac joints known as ankylosing spondylitis. For many years, this condition was considered to affect mostly men, but recently we've learned there is no significant gender difference. Young women who present with morning back stiffness; aching in the lower back that improves as the day progresses; intermittent arthritis of the hip, knee, or shoulder; and limitation of chest wall expansion should be suspected of having ankylosing spondylitis. In some cases, inflammation of the eyes occurs. These people usually have a gene marker called HLA-B27, which can be detected in routine blood testing. Previously treated with painkillers and NSAIDs, ankylosing spondylitis can now be suppressed with biological agents such as etanercept or infliximab.

Chronic tendonitis and bursitis are also common sources of nagging pain that can interrupt sleep, augment central pain, and lead to regional myofascial pain syndromes. This is particularly true when chronic bursitis affects the hip or the shoulder. A tendon is a tensile structure that connects muscle to bone and is sometimes subject to injury or overuse. A bursa is a smooth, fluid-filled sac that sits above a bony prominence in order to reduce the friction of overlying tendons and muscles. Tendons and bursae, when painful or inflamed, can respond to simple rest and ice. Otherwise, this problem is quickly addressed by a well-placed cortisone injection to the painful spot. Other conservative measures such as physical therapy, chiropractic, or acupuncture can be helpful, too. Any good caregiver should be able to ask the right questions and find the typical physical findings on examination that should lead to timely treatment.

Among the inflammatory autoimmune diseases, the one most prevalent in women with fibromyalgia is systemic lupus erythematosus, better known as lupus.

The 1997 Revised American College of
——————— **Rheumatology (ACR) Criteria for Systemic Lupus** ———————

1. Malar rash (flat or raised redness around the nose and the cheeks)

2. Discoid rash (patches of scarring or altered pigmentation)

3. Photosensitivity (a skin rash in response to sunlight)

4. Oral ulcers (usually painless)

5. Arthritis

6. Serositis (noninfectious pleurisy or pericarditis)

7. Kidney involvement

8. Neurological disorder (seizures, delirium)

9. Hematological problems (anemia, low white blood cell count, low platelets)

10. Immune disorder (anti–double stranded DNA antibodies, anti-Smith, a false-positive test for syphilis, positive lupus anticoagulant, or antibodies to cardiolipin)

11. Positive ANA (antinuclear antibody)

The presence of at least four of eleven criteria satisfy a diagnosis of lupus.

Connections between Fibromyalgia and Lupus

There is an interesting overlap in the demographic between lupus and fibromyalgia affecting women of childbearing age. Both diseases are affected by hormonal manipulation, and both are exacerbated by stress, infection, or physical trauma. Obviously, both fibromyalgia and lupus are strongly associated with pain and fatigue; in fact, up to 30 percent of women with lupus also develop fibromyalgia at some point along the way. Left untreated, smoldering lupus can contribute to pain and fatigue and invite a flare-up of fibromyalgia, so its proper treatment can significantly reduce the risk of fibromyalgia.

Other Related Disorders

Not only is the overlap between lupus and fibromyalgia common, but there can be other conditions that can mimic or coexist with fibromyalgia. These situations make diagnosis a little more difficult.

Endocrine Disorders

Several conditions don't necessarily generate pain on their own but can perpetuate the symptoms of fibromyalgia. A common correlate is thyroid dysregulation—either by hyperthyroidism or hypothyroidism. The imbalance of thyroid hormone can be driven by autoimmune thyroid disease, a benign thyroid adenoma, or a thyroid gland that makes too much or not enough thyroid hormone. It can lead to chronic symptoms of lethargy, changes in body weight, hot or cold intolerance, carpal tunnel symptoms, ankle swelling, muscle weakness, tingling, palpitations, and changes in personality. These symptoms overlap with fibromyalgia syndrome and can be confusing to sort out. The key is to suspect thyroid disease and screen properly with baseline blood work, because in just about every case the symptoms of thyroid dysregulation are treatable. Other endocrine imbalances, such as abnormal growth hormone, steroid hormones, testosterone, and prolactin levels, can lead to fibromyalgia symptoms and should be screened for completeness if clinically suspected.

Also under the umbrella of endocrine imbalance is morbid obesity. This problem is increasing in the United States and is relevant to people with fibromyalgia. For several reasons, obesity is correlated with sleep disorders that include **sleep apnea**, respiratory drive, and restless leg syndrome (see chapter 4 for more details). It has been shown that the correction of sleep disorders can promote weight loss due to favorable effects on the brain (the appetite center), and the loss of weight can improve one's ability to sleep. In some cases, morbid obesity is linked to a behavioral eating disorder, which predisposes to metabolic syndrome and the complications of heart disease. This overlap is being described as **TEDIOUS syndrome** (traumatic eating disorders in obese uncomfortable subjects) and is a correctable problem within the sphere of fibromyalgia. For this reason, an ideal body weight is always one of the goals of fibromyalgia treatment.

Conditions Associated with Fibromyalgia

Lupus

Sjögren's syndrome

Thyroid imbalance

Growth hormone deficiency

Lyme disease

Hepatitis C infection

Obesity

These conditions do not merely mimic the symptoms of fibromyalgia, but they occur at a greater frequency among people who have fibromyalgia.

Infections

In certain areas of the United States, particularly the Northeast, Lyme disease has been associated with the symptoms of fibromyalgia. Caused by the inoculation of a spirochete infection after the bite of the deer tick, Lyme disease is the most common tick-borne infection in the country. It causes a brief ringlike rash or a summer flulike illness that sometimes goes unnoticed but is quite treatable with antibiotics. The untreated disease can result in chronic manifestations such as arthritis or neurological disease. Treated or not, Lyme disease can lead to a phenomenon known as post-Lyme syndrome, which resembles fibromyalgia in many ways—tiredness, muscle aches, lack of concentration, headaches, and more.

There is still controversy about the proper approach to treating post-Lyme syndrome. Some doctors and patient advocates feel that a lengthy course of intravenous antibiotics is indicated, although most studies have shown that symptoms improve only marginally. Still, it would seem reasonable to offer antibiotics to anyone who has a positive blood test for Lyme disease and who has not previously received a course of therapy. If the blood tests are repeatedly negative and the person has already gotten the proper amount of antibiotics, the benefits of another lengthy and costly course of intravenous antibiotics become questionable. In such cases, the treatment of residual fibromyalgia symptoms should be approached supportively.

Another infection that overlaps with (and sometimes causes) the symptoms of fibromyalgia is hepatitis C. It is quite prevalent in the United States, where four million people may be infected with hepatitis C, only half of whom are aware of it. While the liver is the main target of infection, hepatitis C has been known to cause skin rash, lethargy, arthritis, and rarely an inflammatory condition known as vasculitis. Most common of all, 10 to 20 percent of people with hepatitis C develop symptoms of fibromyalgia, particularly diffuse muscular tender point pain. This is quite extraordinary when you consider the numbers alone, that so many people with fibromyalgia may have symptoms that are driven by this infection. The conundrum that doctors find, however, is that the treatment for chronic hepatitis infection these days includes interferon injections, which notoriously produce an exacerbation of fibromyalgia symptoms, particularly depression and muscle aches.

Obesity, Inflammation, and Abnormal Sleep

Despite many decades of searching for a peripheral source of inflammation in people who experience widespread pain, the blood test results and the muscle biopsies invariably returned normal. Thus, the term *fibrositis* was changed to *fibromyalgia* in 1980, in order to remove the stigma or the implication of an inflammatory source of pain.

In recent years, however, the notion of a low-level inflammatory state at the core of fibromyalgia has emerged once more. Researchers have attempted to zero in on the markers of inflammation that might perpetuate pain inside the central nervous system. It has been determined that people with fibromyalgia often have higher levels of a circulating inflammatory cytokine known as **interleukin-6** (IL-6), particularly in individuals with disordered sleep and excessive daytime drowsiness. In fact, higher IL-6 levels expressed during the day correlate with the same kind of fatigue that is seen in other inflammatory states such as the flu, rheumatoid arthritis, and systemic lupus.

Likewise, tumor necrosis factor (TNF-alpha), another inflammatory cytokine seen in higher levels in many inflammatory states, has been found to be elevated in the central nervous systems of people with fibromyalgia, obesity, and disorders of excessive daytime sleepiness. Is there a connection here?

The answer appears to be yes. Research by Dr. Linda Watkins at the University of Colorado in Boulder has brought attention to the role of non-neuronal spinal cord glia (including astrocytes and microglia), the supporting architecture of the central nervous system derived from immune cell lineage that has the ability to generate inflammatory cytokines (IL-1, IL-6, and TNF-alpha). This immune activation may be central in fibromyalgia because it triggers a phenomenon known as "the sickness response," which includes altered sleep, memory, learning, energy, hormone regulation, and pain perception.

Furthermore, the spillover effect of inflammatory cytokines in the central nervous systems of people with central sensitivity has been associated with chronic emotional stress and may result in a wide array of unhealthy metabolic disturbances. Such imbalances may include obesity, diabetes, high blood pressure, and heart disease. Dr. George Chrousos at the National Institutes of Health has written that adipose tissue (body fat) secretes large amounts of IL-6 and TNF-alpha, both of which can perpetuate fibromyalgia and adversely affect health in many ways.

Under such circumstances, obesity can be considered a chronic inflammatory state with many of the same immune, metabolic, and behavioral aspects of fibromyalgia, chronic fatigue, and disordered sleep. Dr. Chrousos and his colleagues have also shown that higher levels of IL-6 correlate not only with excessive visceral fat (high BMI, or body mass index) but also with sleep deprivation and excessive daytime sleepiness.

This fascinating correlation among body weight, poor sleep leading to fatigue, and inflammation may have important implications for the overall picture of fibromyalgia (and its potential causes and treatment). Thus, optimal diet and the restoration of proper sleep may have a profound impact on the recovery of individuals with these problems. For example, in people with behavioral eating disorders, the obesity that results from binge eating leads to a worsening of sleep and increased daytime fatigue, and a vicious cycle ensues (TEDIOUS syndrome). Conversely, a good night's sleep, achieved through one of many possible routes described in chapter 4, results in a normalization of both appetite and energy.

The conditions described in this chapter represent a few of the potential pain generators that can worsen the central pain of fibromyalgia. Part II of this book will cover the relevant treatment issues. Ultimately, restoring central balance requires the eradication of chronic pain generators, a major part of the treatment program that lies ahead. It can be confusing to determine the source of your pain, especially in fibromyalgia where the pain is diffuse and everywhere. Yet you must become an active participant in your recovery and do some detective work to help your physician figure out where your pain generators are. You might keep a journal, recording how you feel in the morning, later in the day, and at night, and where you feel pain. Does it move to different parts of your body or seem to concentrate in your lower back and hips? Recovery is a team effort that includes your physician and other care providers, and the more research you do, the more specific and articulate you can be about sources of pain, and the sooner you will learn how to manage your own health.

4

Sleep Matters

A proper night's sleep is crucial to recovering from fibromyalgia, yet many people with fibromyalgia continue to wake up each morning feeling unrefreshed and out of sorts. Why does this happen? And what is the link between good health and a good night's sleep?

There are two important things to remember about sleep:

1. Sleep is not merely the opposite of wakefulness; it is an important part of a healthy and complete day.

2. Sleep is not simply the deactivation of the brain's arousal centers; it is the vital and successful stimulation of the brain's sleep center.

Sleep disorders have become the subject of fascinating research in the sleep lab, where modern diagnostics have demonstrated serious abnormalities in people with fibromyalgia. **Alpha-wave intrusion** is common (faster waves that intrude into the slower waves of restful sleep), while other issues such as basic anxiety, depression, restless leg syndrome, and airway obstruction (sleep apnea) come into play. In many cases, a specific treatment can be tailored to the individual, and the ideal solution to finding a good night's sleep does not necessarily require medication. Some people with fibromyalgia share bedrooms with partners who snore, while others awaken to crying babies or noisy neighbors. Some are short sleepers by nature, and others experience fragmented sleep due to post-traumatic stress.

--- **The Frustration of a Sleepless Night** ---

It's 3:00 A.M., and you have to get up for work at 6:30. You did everything right last night—ate early, avoided caffeine, and went to bed on time. But every time you dozed off for an hour or so, you ended up wide awake again, turning over and over in bed, rearranging the covers, plumping the pillows, even counting sheep. None of it worked, and the frustration of knowing that your morning is only a few hours away just makes it worse.

Most of you don't have to imagine this because you live it. If you have fibromyalgia, with the usual aches and pains and unrelenting fatigue, you might ask, "Which came first, the chicken or the egg?" The sleeplessness or the fatigue? The pain or the restless sleep?

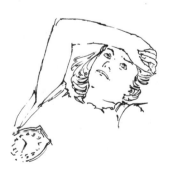

Insomnia is not just a symptom of fibromyalgia; it perpetuates the pain, fatigue, irritability, and poor concentration so commonly seen.

The sad truth is that far too many people with fibromyalgia lack the one essential requirement for sleep, which is peace of mind. For this reason, before accepting a temporary fix such as a sleeping pill or an antidepressant, we should take a step back and search for the missing piece of the puzzle—the unresolved dilemma that might be interfering with restful sleep.

For many of us, there is an occasional bad night, something that keeps us awake before we eventually settle back into a normal routine and a full night's sleep. For other people, the delicate **circadian rhythm** is disrupted for months or even years. When the fine balance of sleep and wakefulness gets disconnected for too long, we feel as if a good night's sleep will take forever to return. People who suffer from fibromyalgia understand this all too well and have usually tried one kind of pill or another.

Normal Sleep Cycles

Before considering the abnormalities inherent in people with fibromyalgia, let's take a look at what's normal. Ordinarily, a healthy sleeper passes through five phases of sleep: stages 1 through 4, followed by **REM (rapid eye movement) sleep**. This pattern is repeated roughly five times during the course of a good night's sleep; around 50 percent of the time is spent in stage 2, and 20 percent is spent in REM sleep. The remaining 30 percent is spent in the various other stages.

The body's physical response changes during each stage of sleep. In stage 1, we sleep lightly and can be awakened easily. This is the stage in which we tend to remember fragmented visual images or have sudden muscle contractions (**hypnic myoclonia**), a feeling that we're starting to fall. In stage 2, normal eye movement stops and the brain waves become slower. In stage 3, extremely slow brain waves, or delta waves, begin to appear, interspersed with smaller, faster waves until stage 4, characterized almost exclusively

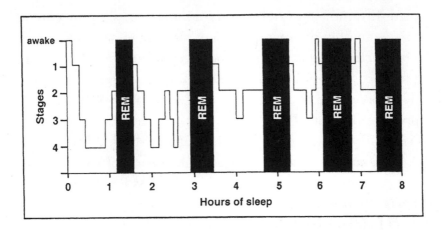

Five cycles of sleep are part of a healthy day. Eighty-five percent of people with fibromyalgia have alpha-wave intrusion, which disrupts slow-wave sleep. In some cases, sleep debt causes premature lapses into REM and further interferes with restorative slow-wave sleep.

by delta waves, the very slow waves of deep sleep. It is during this vital phase of delta sleep that growth hormone is secreted.

REM sleep is quite different from the other stages of sleep. In REM sleep, our breathing becomes somewhat rapid, irregular, and shallow; our eyes jerk rapidly in various directions; our heart rates increase; and blood pressures rise. We usually enter REM sleep about seventy to ninety minutes after falling asleep. A complete sleep cycle takes ninety to a hundred minutes on average. The first sleep cycles contain relatively short REM periods and long periods of deep sleep, and then, as the night progresses, REM sleep periods increase in length while slow-wave, restorative delta sleep decreases. If REM sleep is disrupted, our bodies will deviate from the normal sleep cycle the next time we fall asleep and will slip too quickly into REM sleep. New babies, snoring spouses, barking dogs, and, especially, something on our minds will contribute to this pattern, which ultimately leads to a deprivation of delta sleep.

So, you can see that the circadian rhythm is a finely balanced system within the human body. As children, our sleeping patterns are like smoothly running sports cars, shifting effortlessly through the five cycles of sleep. As adults, however, we are more likely to get out of sync, slip gears, and stall; our ability to sleep falters, and the daily rigors of life become an uncomfortable ride. Why does this happen? Most notably, chronic stress impairs the normal sleep cycle. In other cases, coffee and other caffeine drinks, drugs such as diet pills, and decongestants all stimulate parts of the brain that create insomnia. Many antidepressants suppress REM sleep. Heavy smokers also have reduced amounts of REM sleep and wake up after three or four hours due to nicotine withdrawal. Alcohol, which may facilitate a light sleep, often robs people of REM sleep. Remarkably, laboratory rats deprived of REM sleep will actually die after about two weeks due to a breakdown in their immune systems.

To understand the importance of sleep, consider Rosalie, a new mother, who has been struggling with hourly feedings of her infant. One morning, when the baby is about three months old, Rosalie is out running errands. Already sleep deprived, she suffers a minor whiplash injury when another vehicle abruptly strikes the rear end of her car. The next night, just as she falls asleep, she has a vivid dream of the accident, feels the jolt of the other car hitting her, and is thrown immediately into a hyperalert state. She experiences a feeling of panic and anxiety, and it takes a long time for her to finally relax and fall asleep.

Even though Rosalie suffered no serious injuries in the accident, this does not mean there will be no repercussions. As a matter of fact, it might be months or even years before she is able to truly relax and sleep soundly. One might ask, if Rosalie is okay, the baby is okay, and the car has already been fixed, what's the problem? Why can't she sleep normally? The answer will be crucial to her recovery, but before we continue with her story, let's take a detour for an in-depth look at the nightly phenomenon of sleep.

Sleep Abnormalities

Rosalie's accident illustrates just one way that fibromyalgia can be triggered in a susceptible person. Examples of such brain trauma can include a physical injury such as whiplash or a concussion or less obvious injuries such as post-traumatic stress, an intense emotional experience, or an illness. If you have a sleep problem and you don't get five cycles of REM sleep each night, you are more predisposed to getting fibromyalgia. Indeed, the majority of people with fibromyalgia have some type of sleep disorder that can be demonstrated by aberrant brain wave patterns, as seen on a test known as the **EEG (electroencephalogram)**.

Normally, when a person is awake, his or her brain waves display a random, low-voltage pattern; then in the drowsy state just prior to sleep, alpha brain waves are emitted at a frequency of 8 to 12 per second. As the person falls asleep, **theta waves** appear at 3 to 7 cycles per second, a pattern known as stage 1 sleep, followed by stage 2 sleep, in which faster **sleep spindles** appear at 12 to 14 cycles per second. After this, an important pattern of restorative deep sleep known as "delta sleep" (stages 3 and 4) produces delta brain waves at a much slower rate of less than 2 cycles per second. As stated earlier, it is during this vital phase of delta sleep that growth hormone is secreted.

The last stage of the sleep cycle known as REM sleep is named for the bizarre rapid eye movements that are typically seen, in which the low-voltage EEG pattern strangely resembles the awakened state (even though most of the body's functions are basically paralyzed). When there is a disruption of the normal cycles of sleep, particularly an intrusion of alpha waves into the restorative delta sleep (as there appears to be in fibromyalgia), the body does not awaken adequately refreshed. For this reason, people who fail to sleep well are more prone to having muscle aches, fatigue, and emotional irritability

The amount of sleep required by the average person varies somewhat, but for most adults it is roughly seven to eight hours. This seven- to eight-hour period is not passive or dormant; it is actually a very active period for the brain, and what goes on during sleep is critically important for our normal functioning and our physical and mental health during the rest of the day. With adequate amounts of deep sleep, particularly during stages 3 and 4, we renew our alertness and energy. On the other hand, a fibromyalgia sufferer with alpha-wave intrusion and restless, nonrestorative sleep will toss and turn, keeping muscles tense and active.

Short Sleepers

People who are "short sleepers" by nature do not require a full eight hours of sleep because they get a sufficient amount of delta (slow-wave) sleep in a condensed amount of time. To illustrate this, a Sleep Quality Ratio can be formulated in the sleep lab.

Sleep Quality Ratio =
Slow-Wave Sleep/Stage 1 Sleep + Wake Time

This ratio permits good-quality sleep in short sleepers if they get sufficient delta sleep, a luxury that is rarely seen in people with fibromyalgia.

Neurotransmitters and Sleep

Since normal sleep and wakefulness are influenced by several essential neurotransmitters in the brain, any food or drug that alters their delicate balance can affect how we sleep. Neurotransmitters control both sleep and wakefulness by acting on groups of neurons in the brain stem (the part of the brain that connects the larger brain to the spinal cord). Some neurotransmitters keep the brain awake, while others tell the brain to go to sleep. For example, the peptide

adenosine is released in the anterior hypothalamus as a signal to go to sleep; the longer a person stays awake, the more adenosine accumulates, and the stronger the message becomes. During restorative sleep, however, the level of adenosine in the brain diminishes until the individual has had enough sleep and wakes up.

--- **The VLPO, or the Sleep Center** ---

One key area controlling the brain's ability to sleep is the ventrolateral preoptic area (VLPO), better known as the sleep center. The VLPO, when stimulated, actually causes sleep. The VLPO is where GABA (gamma-aminobutyric acid) and the peptide **ganalin** are released; they are both inhibitory neurotransmitters that activate sleep. At the same time, the VLPO inhibits the arousal centers of the brain. What are some of the arousal centers of the brain? The HPA axis, which regulates the adrenal gland's release of cortisone, also liberates **orexin** (from the lateral hypothalamus), which regulates the brain's arousal center. The locus ceruleus maintains wakefulness by regulating norepinephrine and **histamine**, both of which are potent stimulants (that's why antihistamines make you sleepy). In the reticular formation of the brain, cholinergic neurons release acetylcholine to maintain arousal. All of the aforementioned exist in an extraordinary balance designed to regulate the sleep cycle, and many external influences can alter the neurotransmitters one way or the other.

THE EFFECTS OF NEUROTRANSMITTERS

Causes Sleep	*Causes Wakefulness*
GABA	Norepinephrine
Ganalin	Histamine
Tryptophan	Acetylcholine
Serotonin	Cortisol

In part II, we'll discuss how medications affect all of the listed neurotransmitters.

Whatever may be causing a decrease in deep sleep among susceptible people, the end result is that fibromyalgia sufferers are being systematically robbed; they remain in a lighter stage of sleep from which they awaken more readily. If delta sleep is disrupted for even one night, people with fibromyalgia do not necessarily follow the normal sleep cycle the next night; instead, they slip more directly into REM sleep and go through extended periods of fatigue until they can make up the sleep deficiency. As they build up bigger and bigger sleep debts, their reaction times, judgment, and other functions become silently impaired, and their pain and fatigue only grow worse.

Linking Fibromyalgia and Sleep

If we accept that fibromyalgia is due to an assault to the central nervous system and the disorder is directly linked to an imbalance of certain neurotransmitters, it's easier to see the link between sleep and fibromyalgia. Sleep gives several key neurons a chance to shut down and repair, but if one's sleep is not restful, the same neurons will become depleted in energy and polluted with the by-products of cellular activity. Ultimately, this type of stress produces an unhealthy environment for the sensitive circuitry of the brain. Frequent arousal, poor sleep quality, and other factors all come into play; in fact, a report in the *Archives of General Psychiatry* found that fewer than four hours of sleep per night is associated with an increased mortality rate.

Second to pain, fatigue and sleep disorders are the primary complaints of fibromyalgia sufferers. Sleep deprivation creates problems with short-term memory, depression, anxiety, poor mood, irritability, low energy, decreased libido, and other symptoms. Interestingly, some people with fibromyalgia assert that they are depressed because of their pain, but less than 40 percent actually have clinical signs of depression. So, one might ask, does the pain cause depression, or does the depression cause pain? And why are both pain and fatigue so clearly amplified by stress under these circumstances? The reality is that they all exist under the larger umbrella of central sensitivity, an important topic discussed in chapter 2, "The Biology of Chronic Stress."

Since depression and pain often coexist, fibromyalgia sufferers tend to receive treatment for both conditions. The tricyclic antidepressants (TCAs), such as **amitriptyline** (Elavil) and **nortriptyline** (Pamelor), are often used in small doses to help fibromyalgia sufferers sleep better, but they can actually suppress restorative sleep. Likewise, the popular antidepressants known as selective serotonin reuptake inhibitors (SSRIs), such as paroxetine (Paxil), fluoxetine (Prozac), and sertraline (Zoloft), can also adversely affect sleep. Regardless, the TCAs and the SSRIs are used by millions of fibromyalgia sufferers who have sleep disturbances.

If we come back to Rosalie for a moment, it's easy to see that her insomnia was triggered by a traumatic event. Long after the car accident, she still had trouble sleeping and had no clue as to why. As she continued to suffer from bouts of insomnia, her primary-care doctor prescribed a variety of sleep aids. She even went through a sleep study, which ruled out sleep apnea, restless leg syndrome, and other physical causes of a sleep problem. The final consensus—see a psychiatrist. As expected, however, the psychiatrist prescribed an antidepressant, which did not solve the problem. What Rosalie's doctors have missed—and this is true of most people with fibromyalgia—is that there is not one simple cure for getting a good night's sleep.

Common Sleep Disorders

Common sleep disorders include sleep apnea, various types of insomnia, **narcolepsy**, and restless leg syndrome. Sleep apnea occurs due to a relaxation of the large muscles at the back of the tongue, causing an obstruction of the airway during sleep. It can be caused by excess body weight; inherent physical characteristics such as a short, thick neck; or nocturnal alcohol consumption. This form of airway obstruction results in a pause of ten to sixty seconds between snores, causing the person with sleep apnea to awaken up to hundreds of times during the night, often with no memory of this happening.

Restless leg syndrome is another common condition, possibly caused by a dopamine imbalance, in which discomfort in the legs during sleep is relieved by moving or stimulating the legs. Such people develop periodic limb movements every twenty to forty seconds while they are unaware that their sleep is disrupted, leaving them feeling fatigued the next day. Another disorder known as narcolepsy is marked by an irresistible need to sleep, a chronic disorder of the brain in which a dysregulation of sleep and wakefulness takes place. Think of it as the intrusion of REM sleep into wakefulness. It isn't very common, but it can be quite serious and can occur at any time in a person's life.

Many other sleep disorders, such as bruxism (grinding the teeth) and **hypersomnia** (excessive daytime sleepiness), can be associated with fibromyalgia. You may have a hunch, from reading these descriptions, what might be causing your own sleeplessness. If it isn't clear to you or your doctor, a sleep study, or **polysomnography**, can help to identify the root of the sleep problem. In a sleep study, a person stays overnight in a sleep lab while technologists monitor muscle movement, heartbeat, eye movement, leg movements, and respiration. A **multiple sleep latency test**, done the following day, can also help to determine whether you are seriously sleep deprived or have slept well enough but still feel sleep deprived.

If we return to Rosalie, the possible solutions to her sleep disorder are myriad and don't necessarily require pharmaceuticals. The choices include guided imagery, yoga, psychotherapy, or whatever might assuage her anxiety about the car accident or her guilt or whatever keeps her from sleeping. On the surface, she may appear to be a well-balanced and healthy person, but her anxiety about the accident was never resolved, and she has remained in a constant state of arousal. It's a form of hypervigilance that occurs after an emotional trauma due to the plasticity of neurons in the most primitive part of the brain (explained in chapter 2). The resulting alpha-wave intrusion is hardly restful for people with insomnia, but it's treatable.

So, you can see that, if Rosalie does nothing more than take a sleeping pill or an antidepressant, she will continue to have insomnia and fibromyalgia because the problem is only being masked. If, however, she can insightfully get to the root of her sleep disorder, it is much more likely that her recovery will be just around the corner.

The bottom line is this: for the nagging insomnia that's so common in fibromyalgia, think *pharmaceuticals* in the short term and *behavioral changes* for the long term. Remember that if you fall

---
The Amygdala

The circuitry around the amygdala, the brain's primitive emotional center, where the fight-or-flight response begins, is highly active in people who are angry, depressed, or incessantly worried. Part of the aim of this book is to determine the most rational methods to find relief. Mindfulness, or meditation, for example, has been shown to block the disturbing signals in the amygdala and restore balance in the prefrontal cortex of the brain. People who meditate experience decreased blood pressure and improved sleep. The documented improvements that have been reached through meditation and the knowledge that the brain generates new neurons throughout adulthood means that we are not destined to be depressed, angry, anxious, or sleepless. We can change.

asleep initially but awaken in the wee hours of the morning, unable to fall back asleep, this is known as "terminal insomnia." This pattern often suggests anxiety or depression (or just having something on your mind), a common occurrence in people with fibromyalgia. Some people know exactly what the sources of their worries are, while others need help in discovering their troubling issues. Pharmaceutical options and specific interventions for the various types of insomnia will be covered in part II of this book.

5

Why Doctors Have Failed

Modern medicine has made quite a few advances during the last fifty years. We have effective vaccines, miracle antibiotics, surgery to replace joints and organs, unprecedented recoveries from cancer and other malignant diseases, and, as a result, many people are living longer, healthier lives. Why, then, must someone with fibromyalgia continue to suffer? It doesn't seem logical that people recover from cancer and heart transplants, yet the aches and pains of fibromyalgia continue to incapacitate people. Why should fibromyalgia remain such a source of frustration?

Fibromyalgia and Western Medicine

There are several reasons for this state of affairs, none of which are mentioned here as criticisms, but to serve as a framework of understanding and hope. Basically, Western doctors trained in **allo-pathic** medicine have relied heavily on prescription drugs and the scientific method (measurable outcomes). Allopathic, or conventional, medicine treats disease with remedies that produce effects different from the disease—for example, antibiotics for bronchitis to clear the bronchial tubes, bringing about the direct opposite bodily reaction as that caused by the illness. This type of pragmatism has worked well for most organic illnesses, such as hypertension or diabetes, but, unfortunately, the syndrome of fibromyalgia is too heterogeneous to be measured by the usual statistical methods. For this reason, the diagnosis and the treatment of fibromyalgia have been a source of controversy. The typical person with fibromyalgia suffers from a range of symptoms, as we previously detailed—depression, insomnia, migraines, irritable bowel, and tender points, for instance. To actually measure the severity of these symptoms, which can wax and wane depending on diet, exercise, stress, and other factors, is too complex. In addition, the patient's inability to articulate all the symptoms might compromise the physician's ability to understand exactly what is happening.

To optimally treat this syndrome would require a loosening of the chains that have shackled both patient and caregiver alike, and would require a greater tolerance on the part of physicians to care for patients with fibromyalgia. It also means more time and attention being given to the needs of people with this condition. Seeing a patient for five to seven minutes, writing a prescription, and setting up a three-month follow-up appointment is hardly effective, yet it is all too familiar a pattern. This is one reason why so many people have flocked to alternative caregivers, where they're more likely to get a compassionate ear and some attention.

On the other side, holistic practitioners such as acupuncturists, naturopaths, herbalists, and chiropractors probably offer more tranquil settings and are more nurturing, but they often lack rigorous training in neurophysiology and medicine in general. Again, the one who suffers from this interdisciplinary vacuum is the person with fibromyalgia. We've heard more in recent years about **integrative medicine,** an attempt to combine the best of both worlds—alternative and allopathic medicine—but how many practitioners have really mastered such diverse thinking? Not many. It is only a well-informed and astute person who can piece together his or her own care program that includes all the right elements.

So we're left with roughly five million people in the United States who have fibromyalgia and have few places to go for help. They put their faith in doctors who seem to have a cure for everything these days, but the sad truth is that too many doctors roll their eyes at the thought of caring for these challenging patients with fibromyalgia. They listen to the complaints of pain and fatigue and record all of the normal blood tests, which invariably lead to prescriptions for analgesics or antidepressants. They describe their fibromyalgia patients as being neurotic, speaking of it among themselves in hushed voices if only to assuage their own sense of failure. Worst of all, they get little gratification from caring for people who return for each follow-up visit feeling no better than before. So who's to blame?

In a recent report from Norway titled, "It Is Hard Work Behaving as a Credible Patient: Encounters between Women with Chronic Pain and Their Doctors," the authors describe accounts of women who are met with skepticism and lack of compassion. They feel rejected, ignored, belittled, and blamed for their conditions. Werner and Malterud go on to expose the frustration and the efforts by women to be believed and taken seriously. Why should a person with fibromyalgia have to do this?

────────────────── **A Complex Ailment** ──────────────────

It is a relatively simple thing to appear in a physician's office with strep throat or an ear infection, explain the symptoms, get a diagnosis, and leave with some sort of solution (usually, a prescription for antibiotics). The fibromyalgia patient knows only too well how different it is to make this office visit, especially before he or she has a diagnosis, and say, "It hurts here, and here, and I'm so tired and depressed." If you are fortunate to have a caring, compassionate physician who also understands enough about fibromyalgia, there may be some progress. For too many patients, however, the opposite is true. There isn't one easy solution, and the physician is frustrated as well, leaving the patient without comfort or a cure.

In one survey of patients with fibromyalgia, nearly 60 percent claimed that their physicians treated them in a way that could be considered insensitive or negative. They also said that other people, including family members, reacted in similar ways when they heard about the symptoms of fibromyalgia. Supportive families are a necessity for people with fibromyalgia, but the reality that certain physicians either don't understand or don't care about treating fibromyalgia patients is an issue of some concern. One patient was met with skepticism every time she talked to her doctor. He suggested that if it wasn't Lyme disease, arthritis, or the flu, then she should begin to "get over it." The implication was that fibromyalgia was "in her head," something that is suggested all too often. It became difficult for this patient to keep a positive attitude and really work on recovery. In a case like this, it is imperative that the patient search for a physician who is not only knowledgeable about fibromyalgia but who is caring and empathic. Getting better depends on your building a support network that will help you in this quest.

Understanding the Concept
of Psychosomatic Illness

The answer for people who want to be taken seriously is complicated; however, the blame for the current state of affairs must be shared if any progress is to be made. We have to take a new look at the term *psychosomatic* and adjust our global connotation of it if real progress is to be made. Our lack of acceptance and understanding of mind-body medicine is where the impasse exists, and a change in our collective attitude will become a milestone, if not the first step toward the fibromyalgia solution. Unfortunately, both patients and physicians alike perceive the term *psychosomatic* to mean something imagined, when the truth is entirely different. *Psychosomatic* is merely a dispassionate term that brings the mind and the body inexorably together—not only to explain the syndrome of fibromyalgia but to navigate a way out. Once this is accepted, we can move forward.

Another important obstacle to good care is the doctor's standard, concrete approach to a patient's complaint of pain, and the way a doctor learns to approach the patient's "chief complaint" in general. Early in the process of becoming a doctor, even before laying hands on a patient, a medical student learns how to solve problems using the deductive reasoning of a detective. It's a time-tested approach that works pretty well in a setting such as the emergency room but not when it comes to dealing with a chronic condition such as fibromyalgia.

Case in point: the patient's chief complaint is pain. Now, every second-year medical student is required to take a course called "Physical Diagnosis," in which the complaint of pain is broken down into seven parameters:

1. Timing
2. Setting

3. Location

4. Quality

5. Quantity

6. Exacerbating and alleviating features

7. Associated manifestations

This standard checklist may be fine for the type of pain associated with a tennis elbow or a peptic ulcer, but when it comes to fibromyalgia, it seems that doctors have been asking the wrong questions. A conversation that might lead to a more productive outcome would include the following:

Describe all of your symptoms and how they affect a typical day.

- Are you sleeping well?
- How do you feel when you awaken in the morning?
- What's happening in your marriage/work/home/relationships?
- What happened (illness, injury, emotional upset) just prior to your feeling this way?
- What kind of traumatic events have occurred at *any time* in your life, including whiplash or another neck or back injury, childhood abuse, marital or sexual abuse, physical or other emotional abuse, bereavement, or other such losses?

These are just a few examples of the questions that should be added to the list when doctors inquire about the standard seven elements of pain. In addition, a good caregiver should always keep the following in mind:

- Listen carefully, thoughtfully, and patiently, even if you're busy.
- Improvise and individualize your approach to the unique patient before you.
- Empathize. Find out where the suffering is coming from.

Another dilemma among modern caregivers is the tunnel vision that is found among practitioners of the different subspecialties. For example, a typical thirty-five-year-old woman with fibromyalgia might present with fatigue and muscular pains, but her diagnosis and treatment will vary widely depending on the type of office she enters, as demonstrated in the chart on the next page.

As illustrated, a caregiver can arrive at the proper diagnosis of fibromyalgia, but the type of treatment that is offered will vary depending on the specialty. There is also a fair chance that a caregiver will do whatever he or she does best—for example, nutrition or acupuncture—but will fail to reach an accurate diagnosis or resolve the primary issue, which is fibromyalgia. It is usually after the diagnosis that patients can create a plan using all the different modalities and begin the course of recovery. In some cases, the decision making occurs with the best of intentions; in other cases, the decisions are driven by ignorance or greed. None of this would happen if there were a more unified approach to treating fibromyalgia.

Another issue, which really isn't the fault of the doctors but deserves mentioning here, is the absence of a suitable animal model to study fibromyalgia. Sad but true for our friends in the animal kingdom, there are well-established animal models for Parkinson's disease, multiple sclerosis, and the hemodynamics of a dog under anesthesia. Yet with fibromyalgia, the experiences of pain and fatigue are highly subjective, fraught with emotional content, and difficult to quantify. Because many fibromyalgia sufferers also begin their search for a cure through traditional channels and are so frequently confused and depressed about the puzzling array of symptoms, physicians lack consistent criteria to make diagnoses—and therefore to come up with clear-cut treatments.

For this reason, most of the newest treatments for fibromyalgia have been developed by trial and error, which is neither practical nor precise in such a heterogeneous population. There must be a

Diagnosis and Treatment

Type of Doctor	Typical Workup	Diagnosis	Treatment
Orthopedist	X-rays, MRI of the spine	Disk disease, cervical sprain	Physical therapy, surgery
Chiropractor	X-rays	Malalignment of vertebrae	Adjustments
Internist	Exam, blood tests	Fibromyalgia (FM), depression, Lyme disease	Antidepressants, analgesics
Pain management	MRI of the neck and back	FM, disk, chronic pain	Epidural steroids
Rehab/Physiatrist	Physical exam, EMG	FM, myofascial pain	Trigger point shots, physical therapy
Acupuncturist	Medical history	Abnormal chi	Acupuncture
Naturopath	Exam, blood tests	FM, candida, stress	Herbs and natural remedies
Rheumatologist	Exam, blood tests	FM, Lyme disease, lupus	NSAIDs, antidepressants

better way to bring suitable treatments for fibromyalgia from bench to bedside. Perhaps this explains why, as this chapter is being written, there is still no FDA-approved treatment for the specific indication of fibromyalgia.

What You Can Do

So, how should a person with fibromyalgia respond to the previously mentioned flaws in the system?

People with fibromyalgia are not different from everyone else. It's difficult to accept painful symptoms that won't go away, and it's not surprising that individuals want to believe that their doctors will find an easy answer, a "magic bullet," that will restore them to normal lives.

The research that will help people recover from fibromyalgia is happening now. We are uncovering clues as to the triggers of the illness, which we mentioned in previous chapters, and how these triggers impact the central nervous system. For every sufferer, it is a different trigger, a slightly different array of symptoms, and a different path to the treatment and the resolution of fibromyalgia.

There is no single pill that will lift someone out of active fibromyalgia and put that person back into his or her former life. The solution requires an adjustment of what we have previously believed about fibromyalgia and then taking a new approach. First, you need to have some comfort level with the doctor. Does he or she seem genuinely interested in what's happening to you? Are you comfortable talking about all sorts of issues? If your doctor flies in quickly with a clipboard and is out again, blithely scattering prescriptions for sleep and pain medications, then he or she probably won't help you get better. You need to have a physician who will listen carefully. The doctor should adapt his or her style, somewhat, to fit your needs.

With that said, it's important to clarify that people cannot look only to their doctors for answers. If you suspect that you have fibromyalgia and you have found a doctor who is trying to help you figure things out, you may also need to do a little soul searching in order to participate in your own recovery. You must look within, and into the past, for causes and be ready and willing to explore the many alternatives that exist.

Also, try to find a physician who is willing to treat you in an integrative way. Don't accept a prescription as the final word, but keep seeking the root of the problems at hand. Explore the variety of holistic treatments that may help. You must take responsibility for your own care and take an active role in finding solutions, in order to navigate a way out of the fibromyalgia dilemma.

PART II

The Solution

6

Making the Correct Diagnosis

Before you undergo any treatment for fibromyalgia, make sure that you're addressing the correct problem. After all, many conditions have symptoms that mimic or overlap with those of fibromyalgia, and it helps to understand the subtle differences among them.

The 1990 American College of Rheumatology diagnostic criteria for fibromyalgia require that a person have a history of symmetrical tender points above and below the waist. At least eleven of eighteen tender points should be determined by digital palpation, which means the application of roughly 4 kg/cm pressure using the fingertips, or pressing until the bed of the fingernail begins to turn white. Note that a tender point is diagnosed when the person describes it as being *painful*, not just tender.

When you've had a history of widespread pain for at least three months, you are considered to have fibromyalgia. This doesn't mean you may not have a second clinical disorder, such as Lyme disease or lupus; it just means that the latter conditions should be treated independently. Likewise, the common associated features of fibromyalgia (insomnia, migraine, irritable bowel, etc.) should also be approached individually—that is, separately from the tender points and fatigue.

The two conditions most commonly confused with fibromyalgia are myofascial pain and chronic fatigue syndrome (CFS). The main distinction between fibromyalgia and myofascial pain is that myofascial pain is more of a local phenomenon (a regional musculoskeletal pain disorder). In other words, myofascial pain may involve only a single muscle group, typically a bulky muscle group on either side of the neck or the lower back, while the muscle pain of fibromyalgia is invariably more widespread. In both conditions, the quality of the pain is described as aching or throbbing, which can lead to confusion when trying to distinguish between fibromyalgia and myofascial pain.

The cause of myofascial pain is unclear, but it appears to arise due to a post-traumatic imbalance that leads to localized tension and a shortening of muscle fibers. The resulting tight band of muscle compresses the underlying sensory nerves, and pain occurs. One of the more common examples of myofascial pain is a whiplash injury, when there is sudden ligament damage to the neck. Since the body's natural tendency is to protect the spinal cord, the acute injury of whiplash is followed by a more insidious spasm around the cervical spine that feels like a tight cervical collar.

The resulting discomfort—the trigger points at the **trapezius** and the **splenius** muscles on either side of the neck—is classic myofascial pain, but it's not fibromyalgia if it's merely localized to the neck.

The chronic myofascial pain of whiplash does lead to fibromyalgia in 20 percent of susceptible people, however, particularly if the pain lasts too long. In such cases, the fibromyalgia that occurs after whiplash—also called reactive FM—is more severe and is quite difficult to eradicate once it's established. This underscores the urgency with which whiplash should be addressed after a car accident—immediately, and preferably by manual therapy.

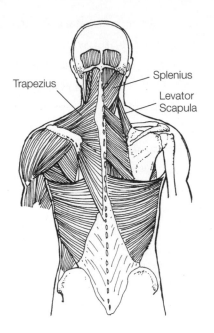

The trapezius and the splenius muscles are particularly vulnerable to whiplash and chronic stress.

Other common causes of myofascial pain include several postural and mechanical problems that can lead to a localized shortening of muscle fibers, such as a leg-length discrepancy, a **pelvic obliquity** (tilting of the pelvis to one side), **scoliosis** of the thoracic or the lumbar spine, and many others. Left untreated, any of the postural abnormalities can cause a chronic myofascial pain syndrome that may lead to fibromyalgia. Understanding the significant differences between the causes of pain is imperative to determining proper treatment. What a physician or another caregiver might do for whiplash or myofascial pain is not necessarily what would be recommended for fibromyalgia.

Chronic fatigue syndrome (CFS) is another condition that is often confused with fibromyalgia since fatigue is a hallmark of both conditions. Sometimes they occur together in the same person, but they are not the same. CFS is more likely a postviral phenomenon that causes debilitating fatigue at the cellular level, whereas the fatigue of fibromyalgia is more likely associated with underlying insomnia, depression, and chronic pain. To illustrate this, CFS is how you feel when you have the flu—exhausted, with some degree of muscle soreness—whereas fibromyalgia is primarily a painful condition that is associated with some degree of fatigue.

The accepted criteria for CFS include unremitting fatigue (exclusive of other causes such as cancer or another chronic illness), plus the following.

SIX OF NINE MINOR SYMPTOMS

Chronic headaches
Migratory joint pains
Unexplained muscle weakness
Sore throat
Painful lymph nodes
Fatigue preventing usual activities
Abrupt onset of symptoms
Fever

TWO OF THREE PHYSICAL FINDINGS

Low-grade fever
Chronic sore throat
Tender lymph nodes of the neck

In addition to the criteria outlined previously, people with CFS often complain of impaired short-term memories, headaches, poor sleep, and postexertion malaise lasting more than twenty-four hours, all of which must sound quite familiar to individuals who suffer from fibromyalgia. Thus, it is easy to confuse CFS with fibromyalgia, and it takes a thoughtful caregiver to distinguish between the two.

Overlapping Medical Conditions

A person who has fibromyalgia may report an underlying medical problem that began just prior to the experience of tender points and fatigue. Naturally, when this occurs, it's tempting to link the illness with the fibromyalgia, even if this is sometimes mere coincidence. The medical conditions that might appear before or during the course of fibromyalgia can be infectious, inflammatory, malignant, endocrine, or traumatic in nature, and each requires prompt and independent treatment by a qualified caregiver (hopefully, one who has added expertise in fibromyalgia).

The relationship of an underlying medical condition to fibromyalgia may be its contribution to chronic pain (rheumatoid arthritis) or central sensitivity (chronic depression), or in some cases the relationship may be obscure (multiple sclerosis). When there is antecedent trauma to the head or the neck, an association with fibromyalgia may seem more obvious but no less daunting to treat.

The real challenge for both patient and caregiver is to sort out people who have primary (no apparent cause) fibromyalgia from the secondary type (such as after whiplash), in order to make sure there is no underlying medical or post-traumatic condition that goes untreated. Your ability, and your doctor's, to recognize when fibromyalgia overlaps with a second problem is crucial to your recovery from both conditions. No doubt, treating one problem and not the other will have a predictably bad outcome; therefore, you must treat the underlying systemic lupus, diabetes, or herniated disk if you're going to regain your health. Equally important is to recognize when a second medical problem (such as high blood pressure or asthma) is mere coincidence and has little impact on the pain of fibromyalgia.

Common medical conditions that may overlap with or exacerbate fibromyalgia include

- Primary depression, anxiety, PTSD, and bipolar disorder
- Systemic lupus and other inflammatory autoimmune diseases such as **scleroderma**, rheumatoid arthritis, and Sjögren's syndrome

- Lyme disease and other postinfectious syndromes such as chronic mono, Epstein-Barr, hepatitis C, HIV disease, and postherpetic neuralgia

- Endocrine disorders such as **Grave's disease, Hashimoto's thyroiditis,** hypothyroidism, hyperparathyroidism, diabetes with neuropathy, acromegaly (excessive growth), and hemochromatosis

- Crohn's disease, a chronic inflammation of the intestine wall

- Multiple sclerosis

- Pancreatic cancer, renal cell carcinoma, metastatic disease, lymphoma, and polycythemia

- Mechanical neck and back disorders, disk problems, scoliosis, spinal stenosis (narrowing of the spine around the spinal cord), and other treatable sources of pain (tendonitis, bursitis, myofascial pain, TMJ syndrome)

Each of the previous conditions must be considered under the right circumstances since any of them may contribute to pain or fatigue, and all of them require treatment. Not uncommonly, the proper treatment of these conditions has a favorable impact on the course of fibromyalgia. Hence, we see the importance of working with a caregiver who is open-minded to the possibilities beyond fibromyalgia.

Finding the Right Caregiver

The right caregiver for a person with fibromyalgia is one who takes the time to listen and care. Beyond that, it is desirable to have a thoughtful physician well versed in the standards of medical care, with additional insight about alternative treatments. Of greatest importance, the caregiver should have a particular interest in and knowledge of fibromyalgia, a positive track record of successfully treating fibromyalgia, and an amiable, unrushed demeanor. Such physicians can be medical doctors, naturopathic physicians, doctors of chiropractic, and other holistic practitioners, as long as they adhere to the basic oath of practice, which is "First, do no harm."

It is the exceptional physician who stops and listens and gives the sufferer an opportunity to express his or her concerns. Unfortunately for people who have fibromyalgia, a lot of work needs to be done in this area. The arena of modern medicine is often rushed and impersonal, and this simply won't work for the fibromyalgia sufferer.

Consider a typical patient, Ellen, coming to her doctor's office for a routine follow-up visit for fibromyalgia. Ellen checks in with a receptionist whose eyes are glued to the computer screen, as she reviews the insurance information. The receptionist hands the insurance card back, and Ellen waits. A nurse calls her in and checks her blood pressure and pulse. The nurse pulls up personal information on the computer, inputting the day's statistics. The physician enters and scans Ellen's details from previous visits. He asks a few cursory questions, and Ellen says nothing has changed, even though she has some questions. The physician quickly listens to her heart and lungs, mentions the need for laboratory testing in four months, and Ellen proceeds to a scheduler who gives her an appointment for four months from that day.

What's wrong with this picture?

Ellen was shy and afraid of saying something silly, and chances are good that she wasn't going to bring up the details of her life under these rushed, impersonal circumstances.

Imagine instead a physician who comes into the room, sits down across from Ellen, and looks at her with warmth, empathy, and undivided attention. The doctor might begin the office visit by asking Ellen how she feels, followed perhaps by questioning what's going on in her life. If there's a problem with work, family, or relationships, the physician might ask Ellen how these things have affected her sleep, her appetite, or her health in general, and how she's handling it. Suddenly, the dynamics have changed; both Ellen and her physician are viewing her "wellness" as a process, and they take the journey of recovery together.

The person who realizes that recovery is not humble submission to the doctor's orders, but a dynamic process, is more likely to find the right caregiver. You are both in this together, which means the physician needs to carefully listen to your complaints. As a patient, however, you also have to participate fully in your recovery. If a physician suggests, for instance, that you have way too much on your agenda and you should take a couple of weeks off and concentrate on your recovery, would you do it? How many of us, faced with a serious medical problem, wouldn't think twice before taking time off from work to stay home and get better? It is just as important when you have fibromyalgia to take your condition seriously. Don't assume that because there isn't one prescribed treatment—such as six weeks of rest for mononucleosis—that you don't need to follow the prescribed care. Like anything else, healing requires patience, understanding, and the right caregiver who wants you to join in the healing process.

If you have been involved in an accident, especially one where you suffered whiplash or another neck or back injury, make sure the mechanical aspects of the injury are being cared for, in addition to the more systemic manifestations of fibromyalgia. If you have been subjected to childhood abuse, marital or sexual abuse, physical or emotional abuse, or have experienced bereavement or a significant loss, you will need a thoughtful caregiver who understands the impact of such events on your current state of health. If you show up at the doctor's office because you ache all over and can't get a good night's sleep, rest assured that a ten-minute visit will get you nowhere. These are some of the things you need to keep in mind when choosing the right caregiver to help you recover from fibromyalgia.

Never let anyone (especially your doctor) tell you that fibromyalgia is a sign of weakness or merely the complaint of a nervous woman. This is just plain rubbish. Too much evidence rests on the side of fibromyalgia being caused by a tangible injury to the central nervous system. Fibromyalgia is not merely a condition to get over, like the flu; in a sense, it's more like morbid obesity because it has definite health-related and emotional underpinnings, has considerable social manifestations, and requires patience and the right multidisciplinary approach in order to achieve a complete recovery.

Like any other chronic condition, fibromyalgia has complex triggers and a variety of symptoms, and it begs for more soul searching and creative solutions than mere prescriptions can provide. This isn't to say that pharmacology doesn't have its place in the treatment of fibromyalgia. Effective pharmacological treatment might relieve the pain, the depression, and the insomnia, giving you a good chance to work on recovery without the stress of such discomfort. Yet it's just as important to look at the primary cause of the problem and the multitude of healthy solutions available. No doubt, traditional pharmacology can ease the pain of fibromyalgia, especially in the short term, but if you understand what perpetuates the symptoms or what triggered the syndrome in the first place, you can also choose from a range of safe and effective holistic remedies. If you ask around, you will find many excellent caregivers who can help you to navigate the path to well-being. As we continue through this book, you'll gather the tools you need to participate in your own recovery.

7

The Ideal Fibromyalgia Workup

Once fibromyalgia is suspected, securing a diagnosis using the 1990 American College of Rheumatology (ACR) criteria is not very difficult. The real challenge, if you want to select the best treatment plan for fibromyalgia, is to determine the driving forces behind it. What laid the foundation for your brain neurochemistry to be susceptible in the first place? What was the inciting event that might have unmasked or triggered the syndrome, and what are the ongoing forces that perpetuate the symptoms of fibromyalgia? Learning the answers to these questions will bring you a step closer to recovery.

Is there an underlying inflammatory condition? A hidden pain generator? An unhealthy atmosphere of chronic stress? Or is it a combination of all of these? You may have some idea already, and if you do, you should bring your suspicions to a thoughtful caregiver.

Sharing this information and finding out more about what may be driving your fibromyalgia is of paramount importance, and as you proceed, try your best to defer to the expert.

Getting the Right Answers

From the doctor's perspective, getting the right answers takes a combination of skills. It requires empathy, an old-fashioned discussion with the patient, a comprehensive physical exam, and the judicious use of modern diagnostic techniques. The tools at your disposal should include a reputable blood laboratory, an imaging center, electrodiagnostic testing, and a certified sleep lab.

In an ideal world, perhaps sometime in the future, we will be able to use an easy, noninvasive method to measure the exact levels of neurotransmitters inside the central nervous system. That way, we could embark on the best available treatments to correct the central imbalances that underlie fibromyalgia. Right now, however, we must use the tools at our disposal to get as close as possible to the answers we need. While some of the newest emerging diagnostic methods may seem futuristic by comparison, the best workup always begins with a personal, one-on-one encounter. High-tech solutions are great, but figuring out this syndrome, which oftentimes comes with depression, insomnia, and plenty of worry, requires a thoughtful dialogue with your caregiver.

The First Encounter

If you are holding this book, chances are good that you may already have a diagnosis of fibromyalgia. If so, you have a choice: you can educate your current doctor about the most recent developments and work with him or her to begin your path to recovery, or you can get another opinion by a recognized fibromyalgia expert. In either situation, a quality encounter with a physician must be honest, unrushed, and friendly.

A successful office visit begins with *you*. If you're still frustrated by prior encounters with physicians, check your anger at the door. Any hard feelings about the failures of the past must be left behind. Be candid. Be smart. Give your doctor a chance to listen. Help yourself by guiding him or her in the right direction. Bring a short list with your questions, and take notes on the doctor's responses.

—————————— **Possible Questions for Your Doctor** ——————————

- Have you had success treating fibromyalgia?
- What is your standard approach to relieving trigger point pain?
- How are you sure it's fibromyalgia?
- If there are medications prescribed, what are the potential side effects?
- What do you recommend in terms of diet and exercise?
- What about time off work?
- How do I explain this to my family?
- How do you feel about holistic or integrated care?

For anyone who would rather see a holistic practitioner, you are encouraged to save these visits for later during the treatment of your fibromyalgia, not during the initial workup. It's probably best to stick with standard allopathic medicine and all of the diagnostic tools at its disposal in order to exclude any underlying medical disease and to document a baseline of good health, if possible. There is little use in treating fibromyalgia solely if you also have diabetes, sleep apnea, or some other condition that affects your health. Don't eliminate the possibility of other factors complicating fibromyalgia. By seeing a regular doctor first, you're not only more likely to discover an unforeseen health problem, but there will be fewer insurance hurdles.

If you're a brand-new patient looking for an explanation for your pain and fatigue, you may want to start with a good internist. If you've already had a workup by an internist, it may be a good time to have your medical records copied so that you can move on to a fibromyalgia specialist. A specialist in the field of fibromyalgia may be a rheumatologist, a physiatrist, or a holistic practitioner.

For the initial consultation, you should bring your most recent medical office notes, lab results, and X-ray reports. Hopefully, you've truncated everything to a maximum of one inch of paperwork. A common mistake made by a new patient is bringing too much information to an initial visit. This results in the new physician spending too much time reading through old records and not enough time with you.

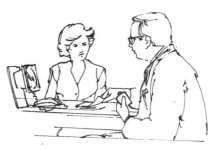

Your visit to a fibromyalgia expert should be relaxed and candid enough to allow a thoughtful exchange of information.

When you call to make an appointment to see the doctor, ask the secretary what time of day the first appointment is usually given. If it's 9 A.M., then that's the time you want to request, even if you must wait a month or more for the appointment. Too many people make a late-afternoon appointment so they can leave early from work, then find themselves in a crowded waiting room competing with emergencies and add-ons. When it's their turn to be seen, they end up settling for a rushed visit with an exhausted doctor. Don't let this happen to you.

The first encounter with the fibromyalgia specialist is the most important of all. It's the foundation upon which a healthy rapport is developed, where precious details of the past are unearthed, and where specific goals are set. During this visit, the basic components of a complete history and physical exam should include the following eleven items:

1. **The chief complaint.** Here the doctor registers your complaint, usually in your own words. "I'm tired and I hurt everywhere."

2. **History of present illness.** This is usually a description of your current symptoms, including all of the relevant information that you may feel pertains to your current symptoms. Your story may begin with an injury, an illness, or an emotional event from many years earlier, and it's included here if *you feel* it should be here. A good doctor will also guide you in this direction. Most crucial are two pieces of information: how you feel right now, and how your health has changed during the recent past.

3. **Past medical history.** These items may be relevant or not, everything from your childhood illnesses and injuries to adult medical problems. It's the doctor's job to sort through this and see what pertains to your current condition. Don't leave something out because you assume it is irrelevant; let the physician decide.

4. **Medication.** A list of your current medications. Here's where the doctor learns about your compliance with taking medications and the chance that some of your symptoms may be due to a drug side effect.

5. **Allergies.** A list of any allergies to medication and the environment.

6. **Family history.** It's helpful to review the medical history of your parents and siblings, followed by your grandparents, aunts, and cousins, since fibromyalgia does tend to run in families. At least half of the women with primary fibromyalgia have a mother or a sister with fibromyalgia. Tell your doctor about other family members who may have thyroid disease, lupus, or neuromuscular disease.

7. **Social history.** This is a glimpse into the personal world of marriage, children, employment, and habits (smoking, alcohol). This gives the doctor an additional understanding of the sources of stress in your life.

8. **Review of systems (ROS).** This is a checklist of many symptoms, complaints, and associated conditions that might bear some relevance to the chief complaint. In some cases, the ROS can overlap with other parts of the interview, although you might describe recent headaches, constipation, and other constitutional complaints that may be helpful to the doctor. This is further illustrated as follows:

COMMON COMPLAINTS

- Fatigue
- Muscle and joint pain (without swelling or focal weakness)
- Headache (migraine or tension)
- Insomnia
- Bloating, constipation, diarrhea (irritable bowel syndrome)
- Discomfort upon urination (**interstitial cystitis**)
- Tingling extremities
- Altered appetite or recent change in body weight
- Exercise intolerance

UNCOMMON COMPLAINTS

Look for medical illness if your tender points are accompanied by any of these:

- Fever
- Chills
- Drenching night sweats
- Any lab abnormalities (anemia, elevated white blood cell

count, altered liver enzymes, altered thyroid function studies, elevated sedimentation rate, positive antinuclear antibodies)

- Persistent weight loss
- Joint swelling
- Skin rash
- Muscle weakness out of proportion to the pain
- Swollen lymph nodes
- Focal neurological deficits
- Temperature or color change in any extremity (can suggest reflex dystrophy, **thrombophlebitis**, or vascular obstruction)
- Abnormal stools that contain blood or mucus
- Any lumps or unexplained growths
- Loss of consciousness, seizures, or delirium

9. **Physical exam.** This is a crucial part of the consultation in which the location and the number of tender points are documented, so that a diagnosis of fibromyalgia can be confirmed by strict ACR criteria. Recall the tender points that should be palpated for completeness: those around the neck and the upper torso, the lower back and the lateral hips, the inner arms and the knees. The number of tender points may amount to as many as eighteen. If you have diffuse touch pain, in addition to the tender points, this is known as allodynea (the misinterpretation of pain from light touch), which may be neuropathic in nature.

All other physical exam abnormalities and pertinent negatives should be documented here. A careful neuromuscular exam is essential to identify the areas of pain, focal weakness, numbness, and temperature or color changes of the extremities. The various causes of arthritis can be found by carefully looking at the pattern of joint involvement, the nail bed changes, the skin, and the lymph nodes.

If there is an underlying source of neck or back pain, in most cases it can be provoked by a good examination. Subtle differences exist between superficial tenderness and deeper pain that can help to distinguish fibromyalgia from other sources of neuromuscular or mechanical pain. Asymmetry of deep tendon reflexes, strength, and sensation can alert the doctor to underlying **nerve compression**, muscle disease, or neuropathy. The following list outlines areas of weakness or numbness affected by nerve compression. Your doctor will consider this if you have regional pain accompanied by other neurological symptoms.

Make sure the pain isn't coming from a localized disk problem or a pinched nerve. Clues can be found on the exam if you have weakness or numbness as follows:

CERVICAL SPINE

Nerve Root	Weakness	Area of Numbness and Tingling
C5	Deltoid	Shoulder and upper arm
C6	Biceps	Thumb and index finger
C7	Triceps	Volar (soft side) forearm
C8	Grasp	Middle and ring fingers

LUMBAR SPINE

Nerve Root	Weakness	Area of Numbness and Tingling
L2-3	Iliopsoas/ hip flexors	Outer hip
L3-4	Quadriceps/ knee extension	Lateral thigh
L4-5	Tibialis/foot up	Shin and top of the foot
L5-S1	Gastrocnemius/ foot down	Calf and sole of the foot

10. **Impression.** This part of the medical report outlines the doctor's suspicions. It can be descriptive in nature (We have a forty-five-year-old woman with chronic diffuse pain and fatigue) or it may be more specific (This patient satisfies the 1990 ACR criteria for fibromyalgia with 16 of 18 symmetrical tender points above and below the waist). A doctor may choose to list the various impressions together (This thirty-seven-year-old woman with lupus now presents with one year of escalating diffuse muscle pains) or the list of impressions may be more distinct in nature (Problem one is muscle pain, problem two is leg weakness). Ultimately, the best impression will arrive at a good unifying explanation for a majority of the complaints.

11. **Plan.** This can be described by the doctor in a narrative form or listed in bullet fashion by outlining how the treatment plan will proceed. A bullet format may look like this:

> Ms. Jones and I had a careful discussion about her fibromyalgia and addressed some of the things that might be contributing to it. I am concerned about the posterior neck pain associated with weakness in the upper extremities. Also, she is overweight with daytime hypersomnolence, which raises the possibility of sleep apnea. I've provided a packet of literature on the subject, and I've ordered the following:
>
> • An MRI scan of the cervical spine is scheduled to rule out a cervical myelopathy or Arnold-Chiari malformation.
>
> • Lab screening today will include a CBC, metabolic profile, sed rate, and thyroid function studies.
>
> • Ms. Jones will continue her efforts with stress reduction and gentle chiropractic adjustments. She will begin a Co-Q10 (coenzyme-Q10) supplement in the

morning, start a light aerobic exercise program as outlined, and will avoid dietary aspartame and petro-
leum-containing food additives.

- I prescribed a low dose of a GABA-enhancing medication each evening. We discussed the potential risks
  and screening required.

- Follow up here next month to discuss test results and
  treatment options.

- If the previous workup is unrevealing and she remains
  symptomatic, a sleep study will be arranged.

In some cases, a comprehensive treatment plan is difficult to
finalize until the diagnostic workup is complete. Therefore, a good
consultation should allow for some flexibility. If there is another
diagnosis that doesn't quite fit the picture of fibromyalgia, the doctor may look for its cause and pursue additional studies.

For example, the complaint of lower-back pain—common in the
primary-care setting—may be due to something other than
fibromyalgia. Most of the time, a good history and a physical exam
will point the doctor in the right direction.

Could It Be Polymyalgia Rheumatica?

If you're over age fifty and you've been given the diagnosis of
fibromyalgia, consider the possibility of **polymyalgia rheumatica
(PMR)**. This prevalent condition affects nearly one in four hundred
women over the age of fifty, and it increases in incidence as we age.
It also shares many of the features of fibromyalgia.

People with PMR usually awaken with morning stiffness that
lasts an hour or more. They describe aching in the neck or shoulder
region and the lower-back and hip region, as well as a deep aching
in the proximal arm or the thighs affecting both sides of the body.
There may be some difficulty getting out of bed, getting out of a

chair, climbing stairs, or raising the arms overhead, due to the stiffness and the aching.

Beyond the symptoms of muscle aching, an astute clinician will
note on the physical exam that the aching of PMR is deep and does
not change very much with palpation of the muscles. This is quite
different from the superficial tender points of fibromyalgia. Another
distinction between PMR and fibromyalgia is found in the blood—
namely, the CBC (complete blood count) and the sedimentation
rate (an indicator of inflammation in the body). People with PMR
usually have mild anemia and elevated "sed" rates, while these tests
are usually normal in fibromyalgia sufferers.

Keep in mind there's often a gray zone, in which a person presents with borderline blood test abnormalities due to lab variability
or concurrent illness. An individual with fibromyalgia may have a
mild anemia for unrelated reasons, while a woman with early PMR
may have a normal hematocrit. Thus, the lab results must be interpreted carefully and with an open mind. A brief trial of **prednisone**
can help to distinguish the two because people with fibromyalgia
feel only a little better with 20 mg of prednisone, while individuals with PMR usually feel considerably better.

Another important aspect of the initial fibromyalgia consultation is the lab work, including blood tests, selected imaging studies, and, when necessary, a polysomnography (sleep study). These
are necessary to exclude other causes of pain and fatigue that can
either mimic or overlap with a diagnosis of fibromyalgia.

Some of the tests are rather basic and inexpensive and should
be part of every fibromyalgia consultation, while others should be
chosen more carefully due to their low yield or high cost. Please
remember that no test is perfect. For example, many people without systemic lupus have a positive antinuclear antibody, and
some people with hypothyroidism have a normal TSH (thyroid
stimulating hormone). Each test result should be interpreted as
only one aspect of the overall picture of health.

LABORATORY SCREENING

Basic: Complete blood count (CBC), metabolic profile (electrolytes, calcium, creatinine, glucose, and liver enzymes), sedimentation rate, C-reactive protein, thyroid function studies, antinuclear antibody (ANA), urinalysis, creatinine kinase (CK), DHEA (dehydroepiandrosterone) level, and vitamin B-12 level.

Optional/targeted: Growth hormone level, cortisol, testosterone, serum protein electrophoresis (test for myeloma), Lyme serology, Epstein-Barr virus titers, hepatitis-C antibody, hemoglobin A-1C (test for diabetes).

Sleep study: If there is significant obesity, excessive snoring, or daytime somnolence.

IMAGING STUDIES

Cervical spine MRI scan (evaluates the posterior columns, disks, and spinal canal and excludes a Chiari malformation).

Brain MRI scan, including functional MRI scan (if one is available near you).

Lumbar MRI scan looking for arthritis, spurs, disk disease, or anything that may encroach upon the spinal cord or the nerve roots.

You need to have a certain comfort level with your fibromyalgia specialist because you don't want to worry about whether symptoms that crop up are part of fibromyalgia or a sign of something else. If you are suffering from pain and fatigue on a fairly regular basis, thus far, then these symptoms can mask another illness that has developed. You and your doctor need to know each other well. When there are deviations from the typical pattern, persistent swollen glands or joint pain, fever, sudden weight loss, rashes, or anything else that isn't typically part of your fibromyalgia symptoms, you need to see your doctor and rule out other conditions. Worrying about new symptoms—or living in fear—is not a positive thing. If you have a good relationship with your physician and can chat about new or unusual symptoms and receive reassurance or any necessary diagnostic tests, your life will be more peaceful.

Also, once you've found a physician with whom you feel truly comfortable, keep on track with routine office visits, regular laboratory work, and medications. Just because you've been diagnosed and have learned all the things you can do (or that the physician can do) doesn't mean that you just sit back and rest easy from then on. Keeping yourself healthy and healing your fibromyalgia means working with the physician to attain the best possible results.

By the time you've finished your initial visit with a fibromyalgia specialist, you should have a pretty good idea of whether the doctor is right for you. Hopefully, you will share good chemistry and really believe that your doctor will be a tireless advocate for you. In most cases, you should be able to detect from the language and the tone of the interview and the consultation notes whether the doctor is being accurate, thoughtful, and empathic. Feel free to request a copy of the notes, not only for your records but to check for the personal warmth and the accuracy of the report. If there are issues you need to discuss at follow-up, don't be shy about mentioning them. Following is a list of signs warning that the new doctor might not be right for you:

The doctor didn't spend enough time with you.

The doctor's assistant recorded all of the relevant information.

The doctor spent too much time filling out a template on a checklist or a computer.

The doctor seemed unfriendly, disinterested, patronizing, or rushed.

The doctor wouldn't or couldn't answer your questions.

The doctor lectured more than listened.

If you feel that your fibromyalgia expert is right for you, congratulations! If, however, your visit was fraught with enough of the negatives in the previous list, consider your options. You may want to give the doctor a second chance and, in a friendly way, lay the groundwork for a more productive relationship. Or, you can move on. But don't stand still. . . . This is your time to get better!

8

Your Way to Recovery

Recovery from fibromyalgia happens every day. It happens in the setting of proper care and because of the determination and the courage of people who have disdain for the syndrome—individuals who simply refuse to give up. Recovery from fibromyalgia reflects the miracle and the durability of the human body. It requires a positive vision, belief in recovery, and sometimes a little good luck. Most of all, recovery happens because of caring partnerships between patients and physicians who tirelessly work together to achieve good health.

As with most other chronic conditions, the causes of fibromyalgia are numerous, and the available treatment options are equally varied. So it stands to reason that the recovery from fibromyalgia must be multifaceted, an integrative approach that includes traditional medicine and holistic care—the best of both worlds.

In fact, the best approach to treating any chronic condition these days is an integrated one—prevention, lifestyle adjustment, medication, and the use of modern technology when necessary. Just as the successful treatment of cancer may include surgery, radiation therapy, chemotherapy, a host of holistic remedies, or a combination thereof, fibromyalgia is also best approached in an integrative way. Just as the recovery from a heart attack requires a combination of urgent care, medication, lifestyle adjustments, stress reduction, proper diet and exercise, and occasionally surgery, the treatment of fibromyalgia also works best when it is interdisciplinary. The best combination for you might include any number of pharmaceuticals, analgesics, chiropractic, nutrition, lifestyle changes, massage, yoga, exercise, and other modalities.

As far as modern medicine is concerned, keep in mind that it's unrealistic to expect that your fibromyalgia will disappear if you use only one medication. If your doctor has prescribed a drug such as amitriptyline or cyclobenzaprine to make fibromyalgia go away, the results may have already been disappointing. The reason, as you've learned in preceding chapters, is that the sources of imbalance inside the central nervous system are varied. Chronic stress of the central nervous system due to physical and emotional trauma, medical illness, and the daily rigors of life are hardly affected by one pill. Most important, the available pharmaceutical agents are likely to affect only one or two neurotransmitters at a time, while more than a dozen key neurotransmitters are out of balance in fibromyalgia. This begs the addition of holistic remedies designed to stimulate your own brain to manufacture more of the necessary neurotransmitters needed for relief (serotonin, dopamine, natural endorphins, GABA, etc.) and to minimize the undesirable neurotransmitters (substance P, nerve growth factors, excitatory amino acids, etc.) until balance is restored.

For this reason, before resorting to a prescription drug, try to adopt a posture of contemplation and patience. Take a little time to plan your recovery, a reasonable period of getting ready to get better.

Recovery is a gradual process. For example, Mary had suffered from fibromyalgia symptoms for five years. When she finally understood what she had and began to plan an effective recovery, she first spent some weeks resting up. She didn't exacerbate her sore muscles. She experimented with things that made her feel better, like a healthier diet, stretching exercises, and meditation. She *believed* that wellness was within her grasp.

She completed any lab work necessary to rule out other conditions and did her own research about fibromyalgia so that she would understand what was happening. One of the hardest things she had to do was take a leave of absence from work. It isn't always easy to make an employer understand that fibromyalgia is real and requires a recovery period just like any other illness. Mary worried that her coworkers would blame her for the extra load that they had to assume and feared that she would be faced with an insurmountable burden of work when she returned. Clearing the air at work before she left helped to resolve some of these issues. Much to her surprise, her coworkers understood and agreed to divide up some of Mary's tasks so that work would continue as usual. Her boss took an empathic approach and encouraged her to do what was necessary to get better. She was a valued employee, he said, and they wanted her back at work in good health.

Mary's husband, fortunately, was also understanding. They held a family council and met with their children and Mary's parents. Everyone agreed to take on more responsibilities at home, giving Mary a reprieve from the usual household duties. Mary's parents were able to spend more time with their grandchildren, and they covered a lot of the preparations for holidays and birthdays so that life continued more or less as normal while Mary recovered.

If Mary had been in an accident and had suffered broken bones, preventing her from climbing stairs, carrying groceries, or driving in carpools, much of this would have happened automatically. Because she had suffered from fibromyalgia for five years, her recovery period would be longer than someone who was diagnosed quickly after onset. Her husband, children, parents, and coworkers were all tired of her "bad" days and her aches and pains, but they rallied when she explained her plan and the necessity of a structured recovery period. After so much suffering, she laid the groundwork for her recovery.

For most people, this period is roughly six to eight weeks, perhaps longer for anyone who has suffered from fibromyalgia for years. During this time, you will begin to reverse the unhealthy tendencies that have hindered your recovery—the negative thoughts, the bad habits, the wrong drugs. When this is done properly, the tender points and the other symptoms of fibromyalgia will unravel just enough to make them vulnerable to treatment.

Getting Ready to Get Better

Before you start any recovery program, follow these eight steps.

1. Get rid of the negative thoughts in your head. Don't be your own worst enemy. If you really believe your fibromyalgia is a fait accompli, the inevitable outcome of the bad luck that has befallen you in this miserable life, it's time to change the direction of your thoughts. Get the negative thoughts out of your head. Negative thinking is not only a wellspring for the symptoms of fibromyalgia but is also the driving force behind many other chronic health conditions. If you're still skeptical about the impact of psychosomatic triggers in fibromyalgia, consider the following:

"I feel a headache coming on."

"I can't face another day of work."

"I'll never be able to sleep tonight."

"How did my life turn out like this?"

Each of these is an example of negative thinking. This habit is hard to
break, but it can be changed with some
determination. Remember, the primitive centers inside the brain predictably
react to abrupt, unwanted stimuli and
cause you (whether you like it or not) to
have heart palpitations, altered breathing, and elevated blood sugar and adrenaline. These symptoms cause the higher
centers of consciousness to respond with
additional feelings of fear, doom, and
vigilance. So, why should it be difficult
to accept that the higher cortical centers
of thinking affect the primitive pathways in a similar fashion? They most
certainly do.

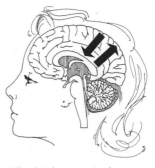

The higher cortical centers
of thinking and the lower
primitive centers of feeling
affect each other. Negative
thoughts have deleterious
effects on sleep, energy, and
the expectation of pain,
while positive thinking is
beneficial to good health.

The expectation of pain has a powerful impact on the interpretation of pain. If a doctor announces just prior to a procedure, "Now
bear with me, this is going to hurt a lot," there is documented proof
via functional MRI scanning that the pain centers of the brain will
become activated and the experience of pain will be amplified. Yes,
indeed, the mind is a powerful tool. The higher cortical centers of
thought and the lower primitive centers of emotion are inseparable.
On a positive note, the thoughts in our heads are relevant not only as
a driving force behind fibromyalgia but as a source of recovery, too.

It is a fact that the human body is directly affected by conscious
behavior. If you're the type of person who feels victimized by your

afflictions, you are more likely to assume the sick role. How you deal with adversity has a profound impact on the direction of your life, and your ability to flood the mind with either positive or negative thoughts will significantly affect your health.

Two women—Elaine and Donna—each have fibromyalgia. Elaine is determined not to let this impact her life too much. Yes, she has incredible pain and suffers from many of the other symptoms of fibromyalgia, but she also realizes that if she doesn't push too hard, if she stops and rests when she is tired, she will have some energy left to go on the next day. She has also explored a range of nutritional supplements and discovered that if she takes magnesium and **SAM-e (S-adenosyl-methionine)**, she will feel better. In addition to that, she learned through a process of experimentation that wheat and aspartame, in any form, resulted in an immediate exacerbation of painful symptoms. Elaine is careful about how she lives her life. Her daily routine includes tai chi, yoga, a diet without wheat, and no excessively long hours at work. She also doesn't talk to everyone about how bad she feels, except for a few people who understand exactly what she's dealing with. And it isn't negative talk, such as, "I just know I can't get through another day like this," but rather, "I need to stop and rest now, and then I'll prepare a simple dinner. I'm not feeling my best today, and I need some time off."

Donna, on the other hand, has controlled her symptoms of fibromyalgia with too many painkillers and antidepressants. She eats what she wants and doesn't believe that tai chi or yoga has any value for her because any exercise makes her "hurt." Not only that, she wakes up every morning and immediately complains to everyone around her about how bad she feels. "I don't think I can do anything today," she says, or, "If you felt like me, you'd want to stay in bed, too."

It's not surprising that Elaine is able to hold down a demanding job. She knows her limits, but she paces herself so that the work gets done. Donna, however, has had to go on disability and depend on other people to take care of her children. She is in a downward spiral that she can't seem to stop.

It's not that either woman suffers from more severe symptoms. Their conditions are quite similar. Yet a positive attitude, an understanding of her limitations, and a willingness to incorporate gentle exercise and a good diet into her life make all the difference for Elaine. Donna's life could be completely different if she adopted this positive attitude—and would be far better if she were willing to explore the possibility of alternative treatments along with her regimen of medications.

In many cases, the way you deal with a health problem is a matter of **learned behavior**, a pattern of coping with illness or adversity. It usually begins in childhood in response to the behavior of our parents. As children, we keenly observe the impact of pain or illness on our parents, and this has a lasting effect on the way we behave later in life. It begins in the cradle for some people, where the concept of mirroring affects the infant as he or she detects the silent messages in a parent's eyes: "Are you okay? Are you sure you're okay? You don't look okay to me. Does she look okay to you? I'm taking you to the doctor."

This type of experience is not unusual, and it lays the groundwork for **maladaptive pain behavior** later in life. Fortunately, aberrant coping skills and negative thinking are examples of behavior that you can change. It takes incredible insight to conquer this type of response, and the effort must begin with a painful journey backward if you are to find your way to optimal health. Ultimately, in the absence of clinical depression, happiness is a choice to be made. Inner peace is a choice, as important as any pill you can take. If you're not convinced, think about it for just a few seconds:

"I feel great today."

"Nothing can hurt me."

The road to wellness is paved with positive affirmations. Toward this end, positive thinking is a skill that can be acquired and practiced. If you feel tense or stressed, you can get into the habit of repelling the tension with good thoughts:

"I'm on top of the world."

"I'm as loose as a goose."

This is just a whimsical example, although if you say it several times (with a smile), you may be surprised to find out how good it feels. You can train yourself to short-circuit the earliest signs of tension this way. Call it self-hypnosis if you like, but it works. The higher command centers of the brain are more rational than the primitive centers are, and we can direct ourselves toward having a better day. In fact, positive affirmations are great while you're taking a shower, driving a car, or pushing the shopping cart through the grocery store—they're far better than negative thoughts. Feeling lucky to be alive can open the door to other positive thoughts.

"That music is so beautiful."

"I'm so happy to be here with you."

For people who cannot find the affirmations within themselves, just being part of a group—whether it's a class of young mothers performing yoga or a gathering of elderly people under the Golden Gate Bridge performing tai chi—has therapeutic benefits. These important connections should not be dismissed when it comes to recovering from fibromyalgia. Surely, before you decide to take a daily medication for anxiety or depression, you should look thoughtfully at your own life and the type of thinking that guides your day and contributes to your mental well-being, or lack thereof.

2. Get rid of the stress in your life (as much as possible).
Okay, so you've decided to get rid of the negative thoughts in your head. Now, however, you're sitting in traffic en route to a job you hate, and when you come home ten hours later to a lazy spouse who doesn't love you anymore, and you're tired and hungry, where on earth are you going to find a positive thought?

This brings us to rule number two—one of the most important parts of a healthy recovery, and one the doctor cannot do for you. Get the stress out of your life. In no uncertain terms, the ravages of stress have been well documented in this book and elsewhere. Stress causes our cells to age prematurely, is associated with heart disease and premature death, and is undoubtedly a factor that perpetuates fibromyalgia. Stress is

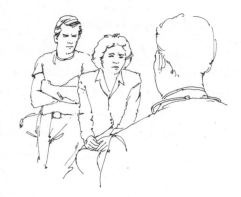

For the best chance of recovery, all sources of constant daily stress must be identified and dealt with. Here, a woman describes her pain to the doctor as her overbearing spouse looks on.

a bad thing, yet too many of us make the mistake of attempting to *thrive* on stress in the modern world. We try to emulate the elite athletes and the seasoned businessmen who seem to feed on stress for success. The truth is that stress is anathema to a proper recovery from fibromyalgia. Your doctor can prescribe the best antistress medications available, but you're just spinning your wheels if you remain in an unhealthy environment of stress. No pain medicine, tranquilizer, or sleeping agent is a substitute for stress reduction.

Figuring out how to modify the stress in your life is an entirely individualized endeavor. Some people may picture their stress reduction as a vacation on an isolated beach in the Caribbean, while

—————————————————— **Getting Rid of Stress** ——————————————————

Find ways to simplify your life by doing the following:

- Cut back on commitments. For instance, think about whether you need so many books, dishes, plants, and so on, or could you streamline things at home so that your house is lower maintenance? Perhaps your children would be just as happy and fulfilled spending one extra evening a week at home doing something with you, rather than engaging in another round of dance, soccer, basketball, or scouting.

- Resolve difficult relationship issues. Harboring resentment or anger creates more stress. Make whatever changes are necessary to minimize stress in this area of your life.

- Look at your work environment. Are there any ways to streamline operations, eliminate time wasters, and delegate to others? Regardless of what your work is, a "can do" attitude and real teamwork will go a long way to simplifying this aspect of your life.

- Make your commute as pleasant as possible with good music or books on tape, or join a stress-reducing carpool.

Chronic stress has been linked to each of these:

- Migraine headaches and tension headaches
- Insomnia
- Panic disorder and depression
- TMJ syndrome
- Irritable bowel syndrome
- Fatigue and poor concentration
- Vestibular complaints and positional lightheadedness
- Atypical chest pain
- Interstitial cystitis and pelvic pain
- Autoimmune disease
- Predisposition to Infection

others may envision time with their grandchildren. Regardless, stress reduction usually requires some type of departure from the daily rigors and expectations that bind us. It requires clarity of thought, forgiveness, and a few practiced skills such as relaxation of the mind and the body. In a study reported in 2004 by Mengshoel, five women who had completely recovered from fibromyalgia were surveyed to determine the most important aspect of their recoveries. In each case, the use of medication was not a significant variable; instead, they all used pain as a warning signal of too much stress in their lives and thereby altered their life goals and everyday obligations. That's remarkable.

3. Get physically healthy. That means doing all of the things you dread. Stop smoking, and minimize your alcohol and caffeine intake. Remove the neurotoxins and the petroleum-based food additives from your diet. Consider your ideal weight, and begin a light aerobic exercise program. No rigorous exercise, weight lifting, or crash diets.

If you plan to stay out of shape and eat whatever you crave, sit around watching TV, smoke cigarettes, and take narcotic pain medications, you're wasting your time. Healing fibromyalgia requires participation on your part, and that means getting healthy first. In fact, there are numerous examples of people with fibromyalgia who have recovered completely without any medication at all, simply because they adhered to several basic lifestyle changes.

First and foremost is your *diet*. If you have a high-calorie diet that's full of animal products, petroleum-based food additives, or dietary neurotoxins such as MSG or aspartame, your recovery will be difficult, if not impossible. Two important studies were published in 2001 describing the success of dietary improvement for people with fibromyalgia. One study reported by Smith and colleagues pointed out the value of removing potential neurotoxins such as MSG and aspartame from the diet. Although the study was small in scope, all four of the women studied had a complete or near-complete resolution of their fibromyalgia symptoms within several months of eliminating these food additives from their diets.

In a second study, Donaldson and colleagues observed thirty people with fibromyalgia who agreed to adhere to a strictly raw vegetarian diet that was devoid of food additives. The study ended seven months later with nineteen of the twenty-seven evaluable patients demonstrating significant improvement, particularly in the quality-of-life scales. These important findings underscore the merits of nonpharmaceutical and holistic interventions for people who are sufficiently motivated to get better.

Diet also implies calories and a thoughtful look at weight control. This goes hand in hand with conditioning, which brings us to the next step on the road to recovery. That's right, it's *exercise*. In nearly every study, a light aerobic exercise program has shown significant benefit for people with fibromyalgia. The popular refrain among individuals who dread any form of exercise is, "I hurt too much to exercise," but if you're serious about getting better, there's really no way around it. Even if you're stuck in a wheelchair, there's an exercise program that's right for you. If you have arthritis of the knees and you can't walk or ride a bike, then you can get into the water. If you have heart or lung disease that prohibits any rigorous exercise, you can still do a reasonable amount of stretching and toning. The combination of stretching, breathing, and relaxation are most evident in practices such as yoga and tai chi, while the more aerobic endeavors have the advantage of cardiovascular conditioning, a measurable rise in endorphin levels, and a favorable effect on sleep. In chapter 10, "Tools for Managing Your Fibromyalgia," you will take a closer look at how alternative therapies can help you.

4. **Get mentally healthy.** Address the emotional underpinnings of your fibromyalgia, your coping skills, your depressed or anxious

mood, your home or work environment, and begin a stress-reduction plan. Get help if you need it.

5. Get all of your pretreatment testing in order. This includes all appropriate blood work, hormone level tests, body imaging of the head and the neck, and a sleep study (if you have problems with obesity, snoring, excessive leg movements at night, or insomnia).

6. Begin to safely reduce the amount of narcotic pain medications if you've been taking them. Narcotics do not address the underlying problem of fibromyalgia.

7. Understand the current thinking regarding fibromyalgia, participate in your own recovery, and partner with a fibromyalgia specialist. Get familiar with the new medications and technological advances that have recently become available, and consider the ones that might be right for you.

8. Expect success. Visualize it.

Choosing the Best Treatment Options

It's a good idea to familiarize yourself with the current available treatments for fibromyalgia, including those that are just on the horizon. You may already have a preference for pharmaceutical treatment versus nonpharmaceutical treatment. In either case, try your best to be open-minded about all of the options. Keep in mind that no particular approach works for everyone, and the choice of treatment made by you and your doctor should be tailored specifically to you.

- Make sure that fibromyalgia is the correct diagnosis.
- Find a caregiver with a successful track record of treating fibromyalgia.
- Be patient—healing takes time—but treat fibromyalgia now.

- Be positive—expect a full recovery.
- Be honest—accept the underlying emotional triggers.
- Expose the pain generators.
- Avoid treatments that don't work.
- Make restorative sleep a priority.
- Reboot: shut down for a complete rest if necessary.
- Find comfort and balance through proper diet and lifestyle.

9

New Treatments on the Horizon

Typically, an individual with fibromyalgia has received prescriptions for pain relief, antidepressants, and muscle relaxants. Any one of these medications may help with some fibromyalgia symptoms, but each drug also comes with its own side effects and risk factors. What good is it to be free of pain if you're sedated and groggy and unable to function to the best of your ability? Finding the right combination of muscle relaxants and antidepressants that doesn't leave you feeling drugged or sleepy can be a daunting task. A long-term reliance on pharmaceuticals alone does not bode well for the average person. While earlier treatments of fibromyalgia relied heavily on medications, and we'll address the topic in this chapter, it's encouraging to note that many alternative treatments are available today.

Migraine and Tension Headaches

Most headaches result from either migraines or tension, although tension headaches are caused by muscle contraction, and migraines are attributed to vascular sensitivity. Sometimes a headache can be caused by both. Generally, a headache is not serious, but it is a major inconvenience for the sufferer with fibromyalgia. If the headache is caused by tension, it is often felt above the eyes at the forehead or at the back of the head and neck, it is usually not one-sided, it can last for long periods of time, and it can begin at any time of the day.

Migraines, on the other hand, are characteristically only on one side at a time but may involve the entire head. The pain is throbbing in nature, develops in the morning, and becomes worse. The attack may continue for hours but usually doesn't last more than a few days.

Although headaches can be triggered by a variety of factors, we know that stress for the person with fibromyalgia can have a significant impact on health. If headaches are an issue, avoid stressful situations as much as possible. Rest with your eyes closed, or try relaxation or meditation techniques to achieve relief. A massage or heat applied to the back of the upper neck is useful for tension headaches.

The average tension headache can be relieved by aspirin, naproxen (Aleve), or other combinations of medications. For migraines, certain prescription medications like Midrin and suma-triptan are helpful.

If you find yourself using pain medications more than two days a week, just for headaches, you may be experiencing rebound headaches caused by a cycle of using these medications. Pain pills, including over-the-counter drugs, muscle relaxants, and decongestants, all can cause this pattern. If you think this may be happening to you, even if the headache is not your most serious symptom, it's a good idea to consult your physician. In the greater scheme of things, the headache may not be your most painful symptom (or maybe it is!), but it can impact your quality of life just like the rest of your aches and pains, so you want to find the most effective way to deal with it.

Medications

Until now, the mainstay of drug treatment for fibromyalgia has been disappointing. A few drugs are listed here for completeness, and many readers have tried some of them already. Several medications have been added to the list because of their potential as adjunctive treatments for fibromyalgia. Five reasonable disclaimers to consider are as follows:

1. Each medication on the list has been shown in at least one clinical trial to be beneficial for the symptoms of fibromyalgia.

2. The medications listed are not necessarily FDA approved for the specific indication of fibromyalgia.

3. Although listed here, no particular medication can be recommended without knowing the details of the case in question.

4. The final chapter of the book gives several examples of how these medications can be applied, based on the origins of fibromyalgia, including post-trauma, postillness, or stress-induced.

5. Any medication has the potential to cause side effects, especially if the dosage is too high or if there is a drug-drug interaction.

Medication Options

Category	Generic Name (Brand Name)	Mode of Action
Neuropathic	Pregabalin (Lyrica)	Alpha-2 delta receptor blocker
	Duloxetine (Cymbalta)	Dual uptake inhibitor (SNRI*)
	Milnacipran	Dual uptake inhibitor (SNRI*)
	Topiramate (Topamax)	Sodium channels and GABA
Best at night	Pramipexole (Mirapex)	Dopamine-3 receptor agonist
	Tiagabine (Gabatril)	GABA-reuptake inhibitor[†]
	Cyclobenzaprine (Flexeril)	
	Amitriptyline (Elavil)	Tricyclic antidepressants
	Nortriptyline	
	Doxepin	
	Trazodone	
Sleep agents	**Eszopiclone** (Lunesta)	
	Zolpidem (Ambien)	Interacts with GABA-BZ complex
	Ramelteon (Rozerem)	Activates melatonin receptors
	Sodium oxybate (Xyrem)	Synthetic form of GHB
	Diazepam (Valium)	
	Alprazolam (Xanax)	
	Clonazepam (Klonopin)	
NMDA inhibitors	**Dextromethorphan**	
	Memantine (Namenda)	
	Ketamine	
Hormonal treatment	(Best if baseline levels are low or imbalance is strongly suspected)	
	Growth hormone	
	Testosterone	
	DHEA	
	Thyroid replacement hormone	

Opiates	Hydrocodone (Vicodin, Lorcet, Norco)	
	Oxycodone (Percocet, Oxycontin)	
	Morphine (MS Contin, Avinza)	
	Fentanyl (Duragesic patch, Actiq)	
	Meperidine (Demerol)	
	Hydromorphone (Dilaudid)	
NSAIDs‡	Naproxen (Naprosyn, Aleve)	Inhibits prostaglandin
	Ibuprofen (Advil, Motrin)	
	Celecoxib (Celebrex)	Selective COX-2 inhibitor
	Many others: diclofenac, meloxicam, etodolac	
Centrally acting	Tramadol (Ultram)	Mu-opioid receptor agonist
	Tramadol plus acetaminophen (Ultracet)	
Topical	**Lidocaine** patch (Lidoderm)	Local anesthetic
	Capsaisin (Zostrix)	Depletes substance P from neurons
	Topical NSAIDs	

*Serotonin-norepinephrine reuptake inhibitor
†Gamma-aminobutyric acid
‡Nonsteroidal anti-inflammatory drugs

The previous table is just a sampling of available treatments that have been found to be useful for people with fibromyalgia. A few treatments have been left off the table because they've been deemed largely ineffective in the majority of fibromyalgia sufferers.

Ultimately, the choices you make should reflect your most troubling underlying symptoms. If your sleep is interrupted by leg cramps, you might find that pramipexole is a good choice—not necessarily to treat the entire condition but as a useful adjunct. If you're disturbed by a sense of burning or tingling in the extremities, you might consider an alpha-2 delta receptor blocker. If there is a component of depression, you might benefit from a dual-uptake inhibitor of serotonin and norepinephrine.

This is a growing trend; an increasing amount of attention is being paid to the use of a balanced approach when treating fibromyalgia. Some people feel that the goal of balance within the central nervous system is best attained with a low dose of combined treatments. Among the pharmaceutical treatments listed previously, several deserve specific mention here. They are relatively new and are part of a desired approach to the balanced treatment of fibromyalgia.

Pregabalin

The membrane stabilizer and anticonvulsant pregabalin (Lyrica) has demonstrated effectiveness in treating the symptoms of fibromyalgia. In a randomized, placebo-controlled study of more than five hundred volunteers with fibromyalgia, those who took 150 mg of pregabalin three times a day experienced a significant reduction of pain, fatigue, and insomnia when compared to people who took a placebo. Pregabalin's mechanism of action is its blockage of the alpha-2 delta subunit of the voltage-gated calcium channel in the brain and the dorsal horn (the area where information begins to be processed in the central nervous system) of the spinal cord. The result is a reduction in the severity of neuropathic pain. As a membrane stabilizer, pregabalin has a mild inhibitory effect on the central nervous system and can sometimes cause drowsiness or dizziness at higher doses. Therefore, it's advisable to start the first few days of treatment at a lower dose in the evening

SNRIs

The **serotonin-norepinephrine reuptake inhibitors (SNRIs)** duloxetine (Cymbalta) and milnacipran have shown early promise for people who have fibromyalgia. They are basically antidepressants, but they also help to relieve the painful symptoms that commonly accompany depression, including fibromyalgia. Duloxetine has been approved for the treatment of diabetic peripheral neuropathy as well, and it goes without saying that neuropathy, depression, and the central pain of fibromyalgia share many relevant pathways. The SNRIs have been shown in randomized, placebo-controlled trials to provide relief in the tender points and to alleviate the overall pain of fibromyalgia. As with any centrally acting drug that can affect the balance of key neurotransmitters, however, caution must be used when starting this class of drug. En route to discovering its therapeutic dose, you may experience nausea or a woozy feeling if you rapidly increase the dosage. Thus, it's best to start at the lowest possible dose (30 mg or less per day of duloxetine, for example), for a few weeks before considering a dose increase.

One of the most exciting developments in the world of fibromyalgia treatment is the practice of combining one novel medication with another. The idea of using an alpha-2 delta blocker with an SNRI is tempting since they relieve the pain of fibromyalgia via different mechanisms. You should approach this new area of fibromyalgia treatment with cautious optimism. When different classes of drugs are used together, taking a lower overall dosage would seem reasonable.

What about SSRIs?

The popular **selective serotonin reuptake inhibitors (SSRIs)**, which include fluoxetine, paroxetine, and sertraline (Prozac, Paxil, and Zoloft), among others, have enjoyed great success and lifted the spirits of millions of people with depression, OCD (obsessive-compulsive disorder), and panic disorder. So, why aren't they on the list of preferred treatments for fibromyalgia? The answer, although many people with fibromyalgia take these drugs, is that they're barely effective in treating the most troubling symptoms of pain, fatigue, and insomnia. In fact, some SSRIs tend to aggravate insomnia. They may be useful as an adjunctive medication for the underlying mood issues that are so common in society but not for fibromyalgia itself. More than anything, the limitations of SSRIs remind us that fibromyalgia is not simply a deficiency (or an imbalance) of serotonin alone.

Pramipexole

Pramipexole (Mirapex) is a dopamine-3 agonist that belongs in the therapeutic arsenal of fibromyalgia treatments based on its ability to ease the muscular discomfort brought on by restless legs and insomnia. Recall that a healthy balance of dopamine is essential—too little results in neuromuscular rigidity, and too much leads to emotional imbalance. An open study of pramipexole followed twenty-two volunteers over seven months. They all met the criteria for fibromyalgia and were given a gradually increasing dose toward 2 mg of pramipexole at bedtime. At the end of the study, the majority were found to have significant improvements in overall pain, sleep, and quality of life. Further studies are under way.

The goal of ideal dopamine balance makes sense and is most promising for people with fibromyalgia who have nocturnal muscle cramps, restless sleep, and **dysautonomia** (the intermittent weakness and dizziness that occurs in up to 30 percent of fibromyalgia sufferers). There may be a role for combining a dopamine 3 agonist with other types of fibromyalgia agents, as long as the potential for drug-drug interaction is taken into consideration.

Topiramate

Topiramate (Topamax) blocks voltage-dependent sodium channels in the central nervous system and enhances the neuroinhibitory effects of GABA. It is approved for the treatment of seizures and is particularly good at controlling migraine headaches. Since it can be sedating, people who have fibromyalgia and migraine headaches may benefit from topiramate as an adjunctive therapy at night.

Sodium Oxybate

Sodium oxybate (Xyrem) is a synthetic form of GHB (Gamma-hydroxybutyrate). It has gotten some attention in the world of fibromyalgia based on its favorable effects on slow-wave sleep and growth hormone secretion. In a controlled study of twenty-four women with fibromyalgia who were given oxybate (6 grams) or placebo at bedtime, eighteen of the evaluable individuals at one month demonstrated significant improvement with the drug. Beyond its favorable effects on sleep, people who took sodium oxybate had a dramatic reduction in tender point pain. They also experienced less daytime fatigue and better morning alertness.

Oxybate is already approved for use in narcolepsy and should be reserved for only the most challenging fibromyalgia sufferers whose insomnia and fatigue have not responded to other agents. A baseline sleep study and close monitoring for side effects would be reasonable, and it should be prescribed only by physicians with experience in treating sleep disorders. Given the potential for the abuse of GHB (particularly if used with alcohol), sodium oxybate must be administered under strict control. Further studies will be required to determine the long-term benefits and drawbacks of this drug.

Opiate Analgesics

There are more than twenty commercially available opiates, some of which were listed previously. Also known as narcotics, their use in fibromyalgia is not strongly encouraged but is inevitable for people who cannot function otherwise. Opiates such as oxycodone, hydrocodone, and morphine are not part of the long-term fibromyalgia solution; they help to relieve pain temporarily but do not fix the greater problem of central sensitivity. Ultimately, the use of opiates makes the recovery from fibromyalgia more challenging. They deplete the body of naturally occurring endorphins and contribute to withdrawal symptoms when drug levels are low. In the short run, opiates are a necessary source of pain relief for some people. Still, it's probably best not to start them at all. Individuals who have been on narcotics for months or years should try to cautiously taper off them whenever possible. As always, the decision should be tailored to each specific person.

Nonpharmaceutical Treatments for Fibromyalgia

First and foremost among the choices of nonpharmaceutical treatments are the natural, holistic remedies. It goes without saying that lifestyle changes, stress reduction, proper sleep habits, conditioning, and a positive outlook can take you a long way toward recovery. Many of these alternatives will be discussed in greater detail in chapter 10. Your partnership with a fibromyalgia expert is another intangible that will propel your recovery, and one that should not be underestimated. A proper diet is essential to good health and should not contain the toxins mentioned earlier in this chapter.

This brings us to dietary supplements, manual therapies, injection treatments, pain-management techniques, and alternative remedies. There's merit to each of these if it's chosen properly; it's usually best to try the least invasive or least expensive ones first. Also, there are important variables to consider when choosing a manual therapy such as chiropractic or an alternative therapy such as acupuncture—most notably, who's performing it—because these professionals include very talented people who have a great track record of success, as well as other practitioners who are less effective. It's usually best to work with someone who has been personally recommended.

Selected adjunctive treatments for fibromyalgia include the following:

- Dietary supplements: antioxidants (Juice Plus+), coenzyme Q10, ginkgo biloba, **valerian root**, S-adenosyl-methionine (SAM-e), vitamin B complex

- Manual therapy: chiropractic, osteopathic manipulation, physical therapy, myofascial release therapy, massage therapy, reflexology, Reiki

- Trigger point injections

- Acupuncture

- Pain management: epidural steroid injections, facet joint injections, **cryoanalgesia**, implanted neurostimulator device, morphine pump

- Spiritual and mind-body: virtual reality therapy, guided imagery, hypnotherapy, spiritual healing, meditation

- Mind-body relaxation: yoga, tai chi

- Repetitive transcranial magnetic stimulation (rTMS), ultrasound, TENS (transcutaneous electrical nerve stimulation)

Dietary Supplements

Among the many dietary supplements on the shelves of supermarkets and health food stores, only a few can be recommended for fibromyalgia. In most cases, a proper diet is sufficient to maintain good health, but in the world of fibromyalgia a little boost from a dietary supplement can make a difference. Hundreds of supplements are available, and some are quite popular, but only a few are mentioned here. The reason is that much of the enthusiasm behind the direct-to-consumer products for fibromyalgia is based on anecdotes and testimonials, and that's okay for the relatively safe, innocuous, water-soluble products that have little interaction with other medications. The products mentioned have some track record of safety and success in treating fibromyalgia, and their benefits probably outweigh their small risks. They can all be taken in the morning for convenience. Most reasonable for neuromuscular function are coenzyme Q10, vitamin B-complex, and antioxidants. Patience is required because it can take months for a noticeable difference to be realized.

Manual Therapies

The manual therapies listed are all generally safe, and they're most effective under two conditions: when taken early in the course of fibromyalgia, or if there's a discrete, localized pain generator. In such cases, the mobilization and the desensitization of pain in a quadrant of the neck or the lower back can be invaluable. Some people will argue that one technique is better than another, but there's little proof of this. Manual therapy in the hands of a talented caregiver can help to propel recovery from fibromyalgia for many reasons, including an emphasis on posture and spinal alignment, the therapeutic benefit of hands-on therapy, and the regularity with which manual therapy is offered. In a rare case, an enthusiastic practitioner will deliver a manual treatment that's too aggressive, which can temporarily aggravate fibromyalgia. This is more likely among the sufferers who have head-to-toe pain (allodynea and hyperalgesia), and such people are advised to take a gentler route, along with a combination of pharmaceuticals and relaxation techniques.

Trigger Point Injections

Trigger point injections are a useful adjunctive treatment for people with fibromyalgia who are troubled by regional tender points or myofascial pain around the neck and the lower back. Trigger points may be symmetrical or regional, and they can be injected with an anesthetic such as lidocaine, **Xylocaine**, or **bupivacaine**. Some physicians add corticosteroids into the mix, but doing so has never shown much benefit. Others simply use dry-needling, sterile saline injections, or the addition of Sarapin (a nontoxic derivative of the pitcher plant) to the anesthetic. All of these seem to have merit. The theory is to temporarily disrupt a trigger point (an area of muscle shortening due to constant spasm or tension), followed by icing, massage, and stretching the muscle to restore its natural resting length. It's safe and effective and can significantly reduce the complications of referred pain, arm or leg pain, and migraine headache.

Acupuncture

Acupuncture is used all over the world for many health problems, including regional pain. In the United States, caregivers of health can get certified to perform acupuncture, and practitioners in the world of pain management (both holistic and allopathic) have adopted it into their daily practices. There is much anecdotal enthusiasm for acupuncture, although its success has not always held up to the scrutiny of controlled studies. As for its effectiveness in treating fibromyalgia, people with the worst widespread pain, chronic fatigue, and insomnia sometimes complain that acupuncture exacerbates their pain. Fibromyalgia sufferers who appear to respond best to acupuncture are those with mild to moderate pain and those with regional neck or back pain.

Other Pain-Management Techniques

Pain management is a discipline of medicine practiced by an anesthesiologist or a physiatrist who has additional training and certification in invasive procedures designed to relieve pain. Originally trained to treat people with terminal cancer and other intractable sources of mechanical pain (such as a failed back operation or reflex dystrophy), pain-management physicians sometimes take on the challenge of treating fibromyalgia. They have expertise in the use of narcotic medications and thus attract unfortunate people who have failed to improve after standard medical or surgical treatment.

Regarding the subspecialty of pain management, people with fibromyalgia are advised to try something else first. The techniques offered at a pain-management center are reasonable for individuals with tangible sources of neck or back pain (such as a herniated disk or severe arthritis) that might benefit from an epidural or a facet joint steroid injection. Also orchestrated through a pain-management center are the implantation of a spinal neurostimulator device, which administers pulses of electricity to the site of lower-back pain or a morphine pump directed at an inoperable source of pain. These are desperate measures, but in a rare case of fibromyalgia that is driven by an intractable pain generator, these invasive yet effective techniques can make a world of difference.

It helps to be honest with your physician about the severity of your pain. That gives him or her the information that is necessary to do the best for you. In addition to medications, several types of therapy can help to relieve your pain, and these should be explored as useful adjuncts. Physical therapy—stretching and strengthening activities—and low-impact exercise (such as walking, swimming, or biking) can help to reduce the pain. Occupational therapy may teach you how to pace yourself and get through daily tasks without hurting yourself more. Behavioral therapy can reduce your pain,

─────────────────── **Ice Therapy** ───────────────────

If you are relying on pain medications to ease your symptoms, you are taking certain risks. There are always side effects with drugs, even with over-the-counter drugs. You need to learn what these side effects are and understand when your symptoms might change or be impacted by medications that you take. You also need to keep abreast of new alternatives that might alleviate your symptoms without the use of chemicals. One of the simplest ways to get relief from a troublesome ache or pain is with ice therapy. This reduces swelling, numbs pain, decreases muscle spasms, and has no side effects. Just as athletes use ice packs immediately after injuries, you can apply an ice pack to an elbow or a knee, your neck, or your lower back. Try a ziplock bag filled with ice and water, or, in an emergency, a bag of frozen peas. These won't be reusable, but they do the job.

Another good idea is to have on hand commercial ice packs (you can keep a few in the freezer). Instead of reaching for a pain medication, try a few minutes of rest and relaxation with the ice pack applied to your most troublesome spot.

You will want an ice pack that melts slowly, to prevent frostbite; that molds comfortably around areas like the knees; that can be reused; and that is nontoxic. This doesn't mean you can always use ice, especially when your pain is severe, but if you have an opportunity to use ice instead of drugs, take that opportunity. You may find that you can avoid pharmaceuticals except when the need is greatest, and you will therefore reduce the inevitable side effects of drugs.

───

and meditation and yoga might help you to relax and may also decrease stress.

Other lifestyle changes can reduce pain, such as getting a good night's sleep—or as good as possible—and cutting out daytime naps. Smokers should stop smoking, which can actually intensify the sensation of pain in some people.

Warning against Prolotherapy

One aspect of pain management that should not be recommended for people with fibromyalgia is **prolotherapy**. Short for "proliferative therapy," prolotherapy is a controversial form of injection treatment that is based on the assumption that the intentional production of inflammation at a tendon or a ligament insertion will lead to a healing of these areas. The concept is to kick-start the body's own repair mechanisms where there may be loosening of ligament attachments in people who are deemed to have ligament instability, injury, or hypermobility. Candidates are presumed to be people who have postwhiplash pain or sacroiliac dysfunction. Usually performed by a pain-management physician, the injections contain calcium gluconate or dextrose, either of which causes a local area of inflammation. The lasting benefits of prolotherapy are dubious at best, and people with fibromyalgia are advised to try something else. It's expensive, it hurts, and it rarely corrects the underlying problem.

Virtual Reality Therapy

Virtual reality (VR) therapy is a fascinating addition to the world of modern medicine. It is getting attention due to its early success in treating several basic symptoms of fibromyalgia—namely, pain and post-traumatic stress. It has been observed that certain types of pain can be relieved upon introducing a distraction. Burn victims, for example, can wear virtual reality apparatuses over their eyes that immerse them in a three-dimensional world of snowballs and landscapes of ice, while they receive excruciating joint mobilization therapy or dressing changes. The early reports look good. These burn patients aren't just *saying* there's less pain; they really are experiencing less pain, according to functional MRI scanning of the brain.

As far as post-traumatic stress is concerned, there has been some early experience among 9/11 victims who have used VR therapy to relive the horror of the incident in order to conquer the fears that grip them. Virtual reality therapy is a marvel of technology. It has great potential as an adjunctive treatment for fibromyalgia, particularly for people who would benefit most from post-traumatic stress disorder desensitization or pain distraction. The solution for fibromyalgia requires creativity on the part of our current thought leaders, not only via pharmaceuticals but with modern technology, too. Perhaps someday VR will become a fun and interesting way to minimize the symptoms and temporarily escape the discomfort of fibromyalgia.

Repetitive Transcranial Magnetic Stimulation

Repetitive transcranial magnetic stimulation (rTMS) is a modern way of applying microcurrents of electricity to the brain. The device delivers a series of magnetic pulses to the top of the head, which induce a tiny electric current inside the brain. Treatment regimens vary; treatment is usually given over one hour, five days a week for six weeks. So far, transcranial magnetic stimulation has achieved early success in treating people with depression more safely than they can be treated with electroconvulsive therapy. And since rTMS can target other vulnerable parts of the brain such as the limbic system, the thalamus, or the hippocampus, it stands to reason that it has great potential as an adjunctive treatment for fibromyalgia. It may prove most useful with fibromyalgia sufferers who have concomitant depression, tension headache, or TMJ syndrome. Further research will be needed to determine this.

Using Medication and Modern Technology Together

Many potential methods are ineffective alone but work well as part of a combination of treatments for fibromyalgia. This is common in other spheres of medicine such as oncology, rheumatology, and cardiology, in which an illness is best approached from different angles with several medications. Remember, too, that if you know someone who's had success with a particular treatment for fibromyalgia, you may feel optimistic about it, but keep in mind that one success hardly guarantees anything. Since some of the nonpharmaceutical treatments mentioned previously have not been completely tested with fibromyalgia, try to keep an open mind and realistic expectations, and check the relevant Web sites for new information.

10

Tools for Managing Your Fibromyalgia

The onset of fibromyalgia has undoubtedly been a terrible intrusion in your life—a challenge to your physical and emotional well-being. Yet you do have more options now than ever before. In addition to the newest prescription medications and technological advances, there are also ancient holistic treatments with a proven track record of success, plus a few things you can do on your own to speed up your recovery and maintain good health.

Just as there is no single cause of fibromyalgia symptoms, however, there is also no single-pronged approach to treatment. Medications and holistic treatments work, but they must be supplemented. Because fibromyalgia is a complex syndrome, just hearing what other people say about their symptoms—how they feel and what works in their cases—may help you to understand and accept your own specific symptoms. If you've ever experienced a chronic illness or if you've been through pregnancy, childbirth, and motherhood, you know how important it can be to find the support of other people who are experiencing the same things. It's not so much that someone else's experience is the same as yours, but rather that another person can empathize with what you feel. That's what support is all about.

You've already learned that fibromyalgia is not a one-size-fits-all syndrome, and that's why the road to recovery must follow a personalized approach. What works for someone else will not necessarily work for you. This is a good time to educate yourself about fibromyalgia, see what's out there, and be open-minded to trying some of the exciting new treatment options. Attend a support group and see how it feels. There are intimate local support groups and larger urban groups with paid moderators and professional speakers. Either type can provide a unique opportunity to listen to other people who have experienced many of the same symptoms that you have.

In addition to support groups, you can join online groups and chat rooms and sift through others' opinions, as long as you remember that another person's experience may not apply to you. Certainly, you can pick up a few new tips for coping with fibromyalgia, and you can stay aware of cutting-edge developments this way.

Along with online chat groups, many other resources are available on the Internet, including newsletters and Web sites devoted to fibromyalgia. A list of these sites is included at the end of this book. One word of caution: sites that end in .org or .edu tend to be from nonprofit or educational groups, whereas sites that end in .com or .net are more likely to be commercial sites where the agenda might be to sell you something. So be cautious about any information that comes your way. Not all that you read is necessarily true, and some of it may be dangerous or unhelpful. Be a skeptic; ask your doctor and other fibromyalgia sufferers about tempting products or advice before trying it yourself.

In addition to support groups, chat rooms, and informative Internet sites, many organizations are dedicated to educating the public about fibromyalgia. Some of these resources are geared to medical professionals, but many are available to the lay public. Anyone who is interested can learn a great deal from reading the current literature written for both physicians and lay people. Again, these resources are listed at the end of this book. Take advantage of the resources that are available to you, talk to people, and ask questions. Much of your recovery depends on educating yourself and finding new ways to get better.

Exercise

Everyone has a different threshold for exercise and pain. Whenever two people go for a long walk, one may be winded and aching, while the other feels like he or she hasn't had a good workout yet. Your own tolerance for exercise may be different from what you'd experienced before you got fibromyalgia, since most people with fibromyalgia describe some type of exercise intolerance. This, however, does not imply that you shouldn't exercise. Quite the opposite is true, in fact; a light exercise program has been shown time and again to have enduring benefits for people with fibromyalgia. Individuals who exercise have better sleep habits and enjoy higher levels of natural endorphins, not to mention reaping many cardiovascular and musculoskeletal benefits.

If you begin such a program, the key is to start slowly. Immersing yourself too quickly in a rigorous exercise program will cause suffering and will result in a setback. If you're unaccustomed to exercise, you should start with no more than a fifteen-minute walk every other day before working your way up to something more aerobic in nature that will get you to break a sweat or huff and puff. One of the most important things, as you embark on an exercise program, is to warm up with a gradual stretching of the large bulky muscle groups of your legs and torso. This should be done regularly and consistently, even if you're not exercising that day. On an off day, it's great to perform this type of stretching after a hot bath at night. This simple habit keeps you more flexible, decreases pain, and reduces the likelihood of muscle sprains and flare-ups.

When you are comfortable with an exercise program, get a buddy to join you. There is an additional therapeutic value in exercising with a friend. If an exercise trainer suggests a plan for you, make sure that he or she understands the additional limits on exercise inherent in people with fibromyalgia. It's not beneficial to run to the gym and spend two hours pumping iron and jogging on the treadmill. It's simply not part of your recovery. If you were accustomed to rigorous exercise before the onset of fibromyalgia, you may be frustrated by your inability to get back to that level of fitness right away, and you should accept a different approach as you recover. You don't want to exacerbate sore muscles and joints and put yourself totally out of commission for an even longer time.

So, when it comes to gentle exercise or light conditioning, do what feels like a reasonable amount at first. As you gradually increase your level of exercise, taking into account days on which you don't feel well enough, you should be able to maintain a respectable level of fitness. If walking on the treadmill is not right for you, cycling is another option, as is swimming, dancing, or some form of low-impact aerobics. For safety's sake, talk to your physician, try things out, and work up to an exercise regime that feels just right for you.

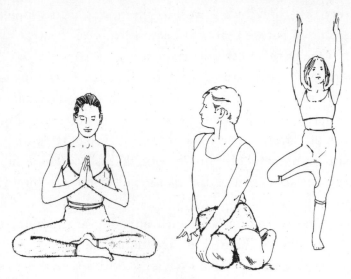

Yoga allows one to relax, breathe, stretch, and tone muscles in a comfortable environment. It can be performed as part of a group or alone in quiet meditation.

Hatha Yoga

Another excellent option for people with fibromyalgia is **hatha yoga**. This meditative, low-impact exercise concentrates on stretching, the strength of holding certain positions, and breathing, followed by relaxation or meditation. The very nature of the exercise is gentle, it puts little physical stress on the body, and it has emotional as well as physical benefits.

Tai Chi

Tai chi combines self-defense techniques with an ancient meditative practice called qigong. It looks like a person is performing a slow graceful dance, not practicing self-defense, but in fact tai chi has a positive effect on health, relieving chronic pain, stress, and depression. Tai chi helps to improve muscular strength, flexibility, stamina,

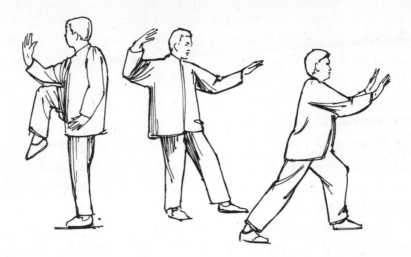

A regular routine of tai chi has been shown to reduce tension, pain, and the symptoms of fibromyalgia.

and cardiovascular fitness. The meditative techniques help to reduce stress and pain.

Practicing tai chi on a regular basis means that simple tasks like carrying groceries, climbing stairs, or doing household chores may become easier and less painful. This seems like a pretty good payoff for some time spent in a gentle, meditative exercise that you can do either alone or with a friend or a group.

Fibromyalgia and Intimacy

It is only logical that if you are not just uncomfortable but in pain, then sex won't be at the top of your list of priorities. This is one difficulty that many people with fibromyalgia have to sort out. If you have a spouse or a partner who supports you in your recovery, then he or she will probably understand when you don't feel well enough to be touched. It is important, however, that your partner's needs are recognized and that there is a clear dialogue about the situation.

This doesn't mean that if you're really in pain, you have to go along with something that will be excruciating—that's clearly not what happens in a good relationship. Yet you must acknowledge each other's needs and find ways to meet those needs.

As a couple, you might discover that there are other ways to satisfy the need for affection and human touch. Sometimes gentle cuddling can be very fulfilling. Experiment with different ways to make each other feel loved and cared for. Perhaps light massage, a luxurious bubble bath, or a candle-lit bedroom can help to lessen the focus on your pain and help you to regain more interest in your partner.

Don't assume that your sex life has to fit some movie industry vision that isn't appropriate for you at this time. You can adapt, improvise, and bring your partner along for the journey. Communication, trust, and understanding will go a long way toward building a healthier relationship that includes your special needs.

Other Physical Therapies

Beyond exercise, you can do a host of things to make yourself feel better. Many fibromyalgia sufferers benefit from massage or bodywork therapists and from visits to a chiropractor or a massage therapist. If you find a massage therapist with whom you feel comfortable, be sure to declare from the start that you have fibromyalgia. That will guide him or her in delivering a massage that doesn't cause additional discomfort, and you just might feel great afterward. A massage combined with a heating pad or warmed stones can be particularly soothing, and although this is not always covered by your insurance plan, it is money well spent by fibromyalgia sufferers.

In addition to relaxing sore muscles, massage therapy is a safe way to relieve stress, pain, and anxiety. It can help you to feel pampered, can release your body's natural painkillers (endorphins), and can result in a state of well-being.

There are several different styles of massage: **shiatsu**, deep connective tissue, Swedish, and an assortment of myofascial release techniques. Shiatsu massage is a traditional Japanese healing method. Instead of utilizing kneading and friction, shiatsu therapists use their fingertips and thumbs to massage and manipulate. Stretching is essential, and this technique works on the body's **acupuncture points**. Deep tissue, as you might suspect, is a more vigorous massage and may be too aggressive for someone with fibromyalgia. Swedish massage is also fairly vigorous, focusing on kneading and friction. Myofascial release technique loosens up the restricted movement of the body's connective tissues and, when done correctly, can give long-lasting results. Any of these techniques might work for you, but discuss your particular concerns with both your physician and the massage therapist before you try anything.

Another highly regarded approach for some people is chiropractic care. Because chiropractors manipulate the soft tissues and the ligaments around the vertebrae, this type of therapy goes right to the core of fibromyalgia. Modern chiropractic care also includes alternative treatments, a plan for stretching and exercise, lifestyle changes, and nutrition. For people with fibromyalgia, a long-term relationship with a good chiropractor can be a very positive thing.

Among the techniques that a chiropractor can use are ultrasound, electromuscle stimulation, massage, and spinal adjustment. Ultrasound uses high-frequency sound waves—as many as a million per second—that create a heat response. This sensation penetrates deep into tissues, relaxing muscle spasms, increasing blood flow, and massaging damaged tissues.

Electromuscle stimulation is done by administering a tiny electrical current into the tissue to reduce pain. People experience a tingling sensation, but the current reduces the sensation of pain, helps to decrease swelling, and promotes good muscle tone.

The chiropractic adjustment is a manual adjustment of areas of the spine that may be out of alignment; it is intended to help restore normal movement. Although there is not a lot of clinical evidence pointing to the success of chiropractic medicine in fibromyalgia, many people swear by it. Chiropractic and massage therapy provide the fibromyalgia sufferer with much-needed pain relief, relaxation therapies, and often the "hands-on" healing and caring that the person may lack in other parts of his or her life. For this reason alone, it can be a useful adjunct to fibromyalgia care. As long as you are comfortable with the massage therapist or the chiropractor and end up feeling better, rather than worse, such therapies can improve your overall health and well-being.

Meditation

Sometimes we dismiss meditation too quickly, thinking that it has to be practiced religiously and continually for any benefit to take place. How, you may wonder, can I meditate when I have a husband, three kids, a dog, and a parakeet to distract me—not to mention ringing phones, neighbors, TV, and other distractions? Well, take meditation down to its most basic level. Consider it a simple exercise that you can do in a few minutes; then let it become a bigger part of your life if it works for you, and if it feels right.

Breathing, which is part of a simple relaxation technique, is fully under your control. You can decide when to breathe in and out. You do it in yoga, and most of the time, you are unaware that you are controlling it. Yet with a little effort, you can make this subconscious process into a conscious act. For this reason, it is an effective part of meditation.

If you can carve out a quiet place for yourself, great. If not, close your bedroom door for a few minutes, and sit up straight with your legs and arms uncrossed. Place your palm over your abdomen so that you can feel your diaphragm move, and breathe in fully. Pause briefly before you exhale. Each time you exhale, count to four. Repeat this simple exercise for four, five, or even ten minutes— however much time you can snatch before you're interrupted.

You should begin to notice your body gradually relaxing and your breathing slowing down. This is what meditation can do for you with so little effort.

Meditation is one of the most ancient practices, but it is completely relevant to the twenty-first century and to fibromyalgia. Because it can help you relax, it offsets the impact of some of the pain and anxiety that you might be feeling. It has been proven to reduce the pain of arthritis and fibromyalgia, as well as to lessen anxiety, stress, and depression. It also eases fatigue and depression, and some research suggests that meditation may help to balance the immune system and help the body resist disease and even heal.

If you thought of meditation as a little "out there," it might be time to revisit the notion. You can use it anywhere and anytime to get focused, calm down, and relax and then, as you practice it, actually improve both your physical and your mental health.

Meditation is now being taught in many places, and its value is endorsed by a number of clinics, hospitals, and physicians. You may even find that your insurance company will cover it, partly because it doesn't require expensive equipment or medical procedures, and the payoff is big.

Meditation is often broken down into two areas: concentration and mindfulness meditation. Concentration helps you to quiet your mind as you repeat a sound or a word or pay conscious attention to your breathing. A mantra, or special saying, can be part of this type of meditation.

Mindfulness meditation, also known as Vipassana meditation, trains you to be aware of the moment. You begin with a single focus, such as how you are breathing, and then gradually expand to include thoughts, emotions, and other sensations. Mindfulness meditation is frequently taught in stress-reduction programs.

Nutrition

Whether you have fibromyalgia or not, nutrition is an important component of how we feel. Yet we often have a love-hate relationship with food: if we lapse into a diet of fast-food burgers and shakes, over time the results will be obvious—weight gain and lethargy. The funny thing is, although we are well aware of this, few of us adhere to a healthy diet all the time. Temptations inevitably pop up. Yep, food is an undeniable pleasure, so it bears repeating: if you have fibromyalgia, a healthy diet is essential not only to your overall health but to your ultimate recovery.

Where does this begin? Eating lean meats, green vegetables, fruits, and whole grains and drinking lots of water and juice is a good plan to follow. Beyond that, people with fibromyalgia can improve their health even more by avoiding certain foods that have been shown to cause problems for individuals with this syndrome or by adding certain things that might be missing in their diets.

For starters, don't eat foods that contain excessive amounts of aspartame or MSG (monosodium glutamate). They have been associated with the excitatory amino acids aspartate and glutamate that are already present in higher levels inside the cerebrospinal fluid of people with fibromyalgia. Certain fibromyalgia sufferers feel better when they avoid aspartame. Ingesting too much aspartame has been associated with additional muscle aching due to its effect on **NMDA (N-methyl-D-aspartate)** receptors that contribute to the amplification of pain.

This doesn't necessarily mean that sugar is better. If you skip diet drinks that contain aspartame and switch to regular soda, you can ingest up to ten teaspoons of sugar in every can. In addition, most types of cola contain phosphates that cause the body to lose calcium, which is not good for your bones. These days, for people who are trying to keep the weight off, there are alternative sugar substitutes other than aspartame. One of these is stevia, an all-natural, no-calorie sweetener made from the leaves of a South American plant. It comes in a powder or a liquid. It has been safely used in Japan and Europe for decades. Another natural, no-cal sweetener is Lo-han, made from a Chinese fruit. Both stevia and Lo-han can be used to sweeten beverages, yogurt, cereal, or anything else. You can also use them for cooking and baking; the one drawback is that they do not "caramelize," as sugar does. Their many benefits outweigh this, however, as they will not raise blood sugar, have no carbohydrates or calories, and have no dangerous side effects.

The other dietary culprit for people with fibromyalgia and other syndromes such as migraine headaches is monosodium glutamate. This food additive has also been associated with the overstimulation of central glutamate receptors that can lead to an exaggerated wind-up effect due to its association with NMDA. We are constantly exposed to MSG as an additive to many of our foods. It makes certain foods taste better and allows manufacturers to get away with lower-quality ingredients. Foods such as soybeans and tomatoes have naturally high levels of free glutamate, which can cause reactions in people who are particularly susceptible. So be careful about the amount of MSG in the foods you eat; you already get enough free glutamate naturally, and there is no need to add more during food preparation.

Foods that are good sources of nutrition for people with fibromyalgia are chicken, fish, turkey, steak, brown rice, and any green vegetables. On the other hand, white rice, flour, processed sugar, and even potatoes are not the best sources of nutrition, so try to limit the quantities of these and focus instead on foods that will provide the most energy and nutrients.

Remember that many people with fibromyalgia have some type of intestinal difficulty. Bacteria in the intestines are natural, but not all these bacteria are good. The "bad" bacteria tend to thrive on things like sugar and wheat flour. The "good" bacteria thrive on green leafy vegetables.

This all sounds very simple, but in the United States, the typical diet is composed of 60 to 70 percent carbohydrates and 5 to 10 percent proteins and minerals. We lose muscle tone and shape, as well as energy and endurance, and have slower metabolisms and less mental focus on such a diet. Both fibromyalgia sufferers and the chronically obese lack the essential building blocks for muscle repair and for fat breakdown.

If you suspect that a particular food is contributing to your fatigue, aches and pains, and lack of energy, eliminate it. Avoid the food for two weeks, and then slowly introduce it back into your diet. Keep a journal, and discuss any significant changes with your physician. People with fibromyalgia tend to suffer from food allergies. If problem foods are identified and eliminated from your diet, you may feel better fairly soon. Changing your diet may not cure fibromyalgia, but it can improve your quality of life.

Your body is struggling to cope with an onslaught of symptoms from fibromyalgia. You need to give it all the help you can. Maintaining a healthy diet and taking care of yourself will help to restore your immunity and relieve your symptoms. We've given a lot of suggestions here that might help, but part of the process is discovering what helps you in particular. It might be eliminating sugar, wheat, or alcohol, but this is different for every person. It doesn't mean starving yourself or cutting out all the things you love; however, making small changes can help you to feel better, improve your immune system, and help you to recover sooner.

Remember to eat a variety of foods in moderation. Don't wait until you are starving and then scramble for something to fill your stomach. Keep healthy snacks on hand. In a pinch, this might prevent you from succumbing to the fast food lure. You can keep a piece of fruit or a healthy snack in your car, your briefcase, or your purse. In your own kitchen, you are even better prepared if you plan ahead. Shop with your needs (not just your desires) in mind. Buy things that will be tasty and nutritious, and, if it suits you better, eat six small meals a day rather than the traditional three meals. This might mean that you don't find yourself starving and fatigued at 5 P.M., with another hour or two to go until dinner.

You can use tasty spices to enhance your meals, rather than relying too heavily on salt or sugar. Keep healthy convenience foods on hand, such as precut vegetables, so that you don't spend a lot of time standing in the kitchen. This might help you on a day when you don't feel well, yet you really need a good meal. Invest in appliances like a food processor, a blender, or an electric can opener to reduce painful, repetitive motions.

Avoid foods that might trigger digestive problems, which may be part of your fibromyalgia symptoms. Heartburn can be triggered by acidic foods—tomato sauce, pizza, spicy foods—and irritable bowel syndrome, common among fibromyalgia sufferers, is exacerbated by any foods that may cause constipation or diarrhea.

Once you have cut out some of the foods that might contribute to your illness, look at what's missing and what you can add. A magnesium deficiency, for instance, is common in people with fibromyalgia. Magnesium is important for the proper functioning of muscles, including the heart, and it relieves muscle spasms and pain. A calcium deficiency can also cause muscle cramps, and calcium supplements should be combined with magnesium.

Essential amino acids and certain essential fatty acids can help to protect against cell damage, and might even reduce pain and fatigue. **Fish oil** contains the essential fatty acids omega-3 EPA and DHA, which are natural anti-inflammatories that can help relieve pain. Vitamins A and E have been shown to enhance the body's immune function, vitamins B12 and B6 work with other B vitamins to provide energy and maintain normal brain function, and vitamin C with bioflavonoids has favorable effects on immune function and cartilage and can increase your energy level.

Another nutritional supplement that has proven helpful for people with fibromyalgia is **proanthocyanidin** (grape seed extract, Pycnogenol), an antioxidant that can protect against degenerative diseases. It also has anti-inflammatory and circulatory benefits.

Some fibromyalgia sufferers have found that adding **lecithin** to their diets is beneficial. This fatlike substance, called a phospholipid, is needed by every cell in the body and is a crucial building block of cell membranes. Lecithin supports the myelin sheath of the nerves similar to the way that insulation enhances the electrical conductivity of a wire. It is best used in combination with B-complex vitamins for people who have neuropathic symptoms (burning, tingling, parasthesia).

In some cases, nutrition in fibromyalgia is a trial-and-error affair: what works for one person may not be perfect for another. Sometimes you need to try an elimination diet to figure out which foods you may be sensitive or allergic to. Evaluate your diet, discuss it with your physician, and make sure that you get all the proper nutrients and vitamins that you need.

Irritable Bowel Syndrome

Irritable bowel syndrome (IBS) is, unfortunately, a very common symptom of fibromyalgia, and one that can affect people in unforeseen ways. It is also known as spastic colon, mucous colitis, spastic colitis, nervous stomach, or irritable colon. There isn't a structural or a biochemical cause, but rather a functional one—in other words, it can't be diagnosed by common techniques such as X-rays or blood tests.

It is basically a disturbance in the interaction between the gut or intestines, the brain, and the autonomic nervous system, which regulates bowel motility. Abdominal pain or discomfort is linked with changes in bowel pattern, such as loose or more frequent bowel movements, diarrhea, or constipation.

We often hear about stress being associated with IBS. Perhaps symptoms of IBS get worse with stress, and in chapter 2, we explored the relationship between stress and other aspects of our health. Our stress response can include subjective feelings, and our bodies consistently respond in automatic ways, often without our being aware. Whenever such stressors and the resultant emotions come into play, our bodies may act in ways that are beyond our control. The limbic system induces a biological response in the body, which includes stimulation of the cardiovascular system (increased blood pressure, heart rate, cardiac output), to prepare the body for the fight-or-flight response. Fear is associated with the inhibition of upper gastrointestinal (GI; stomach and duodenum) contractions and secretions and with stimulation of lower GI (sigmoid colon and rectum) motility and secretions. The former may contribute to a sensation of fullness and lack of appetite, the latter to diarrhea and lower abdominal pain.

This response may have evolved to minimize exposure of the small and the large intestines to ingested food and waste material at a time when all energy is shunted toward the fight-or-flight response. Somehow, when emotions change to anger, the pattern of the upper GI activity is reversed, with the stimulation of gastric contractions and acid secretion.

Unfortunately, humans experience the wear and tear of stress. You may be resilient to this stress. Perhaps you have a good support network, good genes, and so on, and the impact of stress isn't as severe. The chronic effects of stress on the GI tract can be lasting, however. For women, particularly, the increased stress responsiveness, due in part to their nurturing role in life, may create more problems with IBS than it does for men. Studies have also shown that women who suffered certain stressors before age ten, such as loss of the primary caregiver, a distant mother-child relationship, emotional neglect, and physical and verbal or sexual abuse, may be more likely to develop IBS later in life.

Unfortunately, as people begin to understand the stress responses that trigger IBS symptoms, they may also develop anxiety and fear related directly to these symptoms. In other words, you remain in a chronically anxious state because, perhaps, you worry about being close enough to a bathroom or you feel concerned about the onset of symptoms during an important meeting. This is not a small thing to people who suffer from IBS.

Learning to cope with IBS, however—and there are ways to cope—can improve your quality of life. Cognitive and behavioral approaches can be useful. Develop effective coping styles toward life stress and IBS symptoms, and learn to activate mechanisms in the body that oppose the stress response and induce the relaxation response, such as relaxation, breathing exercises, hypnosis, meditation, and moderate but sustained exercise.

Irritable Bladder

Like irritable bowel syndrome, many people with fibromyalgia experience irritable bladder, an equally inconvenient and painful symptom. This is known as interstitial cystitis or painful bladder syndrome. The condition can range from mild to more severe in different people and even in the same person at different times. Some people experience discomfort, pressure, and tenderness in the bladder area. There may be an urgent need to urinate or a need to urinate frequently. Although cystitis will often be diagnosed with the existence of certain bacteria in a culture, irritable bladder may occur without infection. It is also more frequent in women, typical of many of the symptoms of fibromyalgia.

Irritable bladder is generally diagnosed when the presence of infection or cancer has been ruled out. If there is infection, then antibiotics are often the routine course of treatment. If it is irritable bladder and it is a persistent problem, then transcutaneous electrical nerve stimulation (TENS), a technique that is used for other types of fibromyalgia pain, can be very effective. It does seem to help minimize pelvic pain.

Once the pain has been relieved, then gentle stretching exercises and bladder training (creating a schedule and working to maintain it by using relaxation techniques) can be beneficial. If you understand what is happening—chronic discomfort, of course, leads to the anticipation of discomfort and other unpleasant feelings—then you can work to control the symptoms just as you might concentrate on helping yourself to alleviate other types of fibromyalgia pain.

Moving into Wellness

For people with fibromyalgia, recovery always seems like a lengthy process, but be patient. The longer you've been sick, the longer it can take to recuperate. Allow your body the necessary time to heal. It's a process that occurs gradually as your central nervous system finds its proper balance, so don't eagerly overexert yourself in exercise, and don't try too many new things at once. It's quite possible that you will have to take time off work—perhaps weeks or months—a necessary amount of time to eliminate the stress. During this break in your routine, you can spend quality time resting and building up your strength. Your family or your employer should view this as a mandatory recovery period, not unlike the time taken after childbirth or a heart attack. If you are a young mother who is overwhelmed by the demands of small children, you must get some help and find time during the day to rest properly as you recover. Explain to your spouse or your boss that there's nothing more important than your health. Once you take the time to recuperate, you can return to your normal life—or to an even better one.

If your pain was caused by an injury, consider the active pain generators that must be addressed. If your tender points become particularly sore after exercise, understand what your limits are, and find someone who knows how to use his or her hands or the right syringe to alleviate your peripheral tender points. If you're sensitive to certain foods in your diet, remember that sacrificing your health is not worth the sugar, NutraSweet, MSG, wheat, or whatever else might cause a flare-up of your symptoms. Once you have determined the specific triggers that make you hurt, you will learn how to eliminate the pain. Please don't ignore the emotional traumas that leave so many people susceptible to fibromyalgia. Even if you've suffered a traumatic experience long ago, give credence to the wonderful investigative work that can be accomplished by a thoughtful mental health worker, accept the connection between the mind and the body, and find one of the newest techniques to facilitate healing. This can be accomplished in so many ways, and it always begins with an honest, open-minded appraisal of your own mental health.

Finally, it is important to accept that fibromyalgia is not necessarily a permanent condition. If damage has been done to your body and the central nervous system, in many cases the damage can be undone—but it is not a simple process. Recovery requires soul searching and patience, trial and error on the part of both patient and physician, and certain lifestyle adjustments.

There is not one simple way to regain your health. Relief is available for pain, sleep difficulties, and depression, but no treatment is uniformly successful. So if you try something that doesn't work, don't despair. Ultimately, the path to a life free from fibromyalgia requires the series of logical steps described in this book, including available treatments in both conventional and alternative medicine. It means being open to alternatives such as yoga, tai chi, dietary changes, and mind-body medicine.

Educate yourself first about what has happened to your body and then about what can be done to fix it. You must be motivated to get better and be inspired by the vision of a pain-free future. As always, keep your physician informed about any of your plans to begin exercising or taking supplements or to undergo alternative treatments. Make sure your caregivers are empathic, understanding, and available to you, and never give up hope. Countless people have recovered from their ordeal with fibromyalgia, and you can, too.

Love, Humor, and Peace of Mind

No matter which type of fibromyalgia describes yours best (postinjury, postillness, or stress-driven), there are three important themes to remember, all time-tested vehicles to recovery. In no particular order, they are love, humor, and peace of mind.

Love is not only a powerful emotion; it is also a highly effective emollient. It is a temporary antidote to the negative feelings and the stress that often accompany fibromyalgia, and it should never be underestimated as a source of nurturing and healing. Whether giving love, getting love, or making love appeals to you most, the goal is to find it, foster it, and embrace it.

Where is the best place to begin? Not surprisingly, if you want to be loved, you must be willing to love others. It also helps to feel good about yourself, even to love yourself. It requires a willingness to reach out to others with a phone call, a knock on the door, or perhaps just a soft touch on the arm. In some cases, it begins with a short walk across the room toward a spouse or a friend or with a letter written from the heart. Love creates vulnerability and exposure but is generally worth the risk. It's a statement that you do not want to be isolated during your recovery.

This type of connection with others is vital, as real as the pain in your muscles, and is worth trying. For too many people, the absence of love is worse than any vitamin deficiency and far more pernicious. On the other hand, love is inexpensive and widely available if you open your heart and allow it into your life.

The experience of love always begins with an open mind, and this may be a problem for people who have suffered from emotional abuse or PTSD. After all, love requires trust, and a part of yourself may be closed off to others if you've experienced violence, sexual abuse, or neglect in your life. It takes great courage to embark on a healing process that includes trust, acceptance, forgiveness, and a loving connection to others.

Even in the absence of PTSD or such extreme circumstances, it is easy to feel isolated, lonely, or overwhelmed in a modern society. Too often, a busy schedule cuts into quality time with the people you love, but there's something you can do about this. Make your favorite relationships a priority (sooner rather than later), and spend more time doing things that make you happy.

But wait, what about central sensitivity? What about excitatory neurotoxins and NMDA receptors? Isn't there a more sophisticated solution to fibromyalgia than love? Yes, of course, but if a thoughtful discussion includes objective parameters, pain generators, and alpha-intrusion insomnia, one's state of mind is as crucial as any physiological measure. A pain generator is just as likely to be emotional as physical. The alteration of sensory mapping in the central nervous system can be driven by lust, rage, jealousy, or obsession, as well as by fever or concussion. Fragmented sleep might begin with a broken heart as easily as with a broken collar bone. Of all the potential healing effects attributed to one's emotional state, none is more potent than love itself.

You may ask, particularly if you feel unloved, where are you going to find love? The answer begins with loving others—usually, people closest to you—but if not within the walls of your home, then by reaching out. The possibilities are limitless. For some people, it may be an entirely social endeavor; for others, the experience of love may be wholly platonic—a volunteer effort, for example. Or perhaps taking a group trip somewhere—a cruise or a tour. You never know who is waiting out there with similar needs. Even the planning process of such an adventure promotes a healthy flow of hormones and a sense of wellness.

Equally as important as love is humor, the ability to see the lighter side of things. A cheerful attitude and a good sense of humor are the first lines of defense against bad luck, bad genes, cancer, illness, or just a miserable day. On a physiological level, laughter is actually the best medicine; it fosters the healing process of fibromyalgia as well as does any pill in the pharmacy. Fortunately, a good sense of humor doesn't require that you make the jokes as long as you get the joke. Making others laugh is a gift that's hard to come by, but we all have the ability to laugh.

Some people might be thinking, "Hey, wait a minute. Fibromyalgia is no joke, buster." It is, though, when you think about it—if you allow it to be. If you have the nerve to put fibromyalgia in its place.

Actually, humor is nothing new; it's been part of the fabric of healing since the advent of medicine itself. The medical benefits of a good laugh go without saying—increased natural endorphins and serotonin, a stronger immune system, and more. A self-effacing nature has comforted many a beleaguered immigrant, starving nations, and even the privileged few. In each case, the ability to see the lighter side of a bad situation makes a painful journey more bearable.

If you think you're too tired or uncomfortable to tap into the funny side of life, give it a try anyway. Your ability to diffuse some of the pain with a smile or a joke will not only help you feel better but will also comfort people who are concerned about you.

Another key to your recovery is peace of mind. No question about it, in the hectic pace of the modern world there is a distinct shortage of peace of mind, serenity, and tranquillity. And in the world of fibromyalgia there is no substitute for peace of mind, which always translates into better sleep, a reduction of muscle tension, normalization of appetite, and a smoother autonomic nervous system. Peace of mind is the antidote to the "sickness syndrome" driven by chronic stress.

An escalation of stress always seems to hit you when you're most vulnerable and results in an unwanted, persistent activation of both central pain processing and a low-grade inflammatory response inside the central nervous system. Far more insidious than any diagnosis of anxiety or depression is the constant exposure to stress. This unhealthy experience is likely responsible for many cases of central sensitivity seen in the aftermath of prolonged tragedy or illness or in the setting of PTSD. The human body is well equipped to deal with brief periods of stress, and the immune system is primed to fight off brief inflammatory states such as infection or exposure to foreign proteins, but these protective systems begin to break down when faced with a constant exposure to unhealthy stress. Neither the neuroendocrine cascade of hormones nor the sophisticated immune defenses so crucial to our survival as a species hold up very well to this.

The resulting breakdown of immune surveillance and the dysregulation of the HPA axis ultimately create a perfect milieu for fibromyalgia. Most people who are sleep deprived or under considerable stress are unaware that just one more straw will break the camel's back—infection, whiplash, exhaustion—and the cycle of pain begins. This is entirely preventable, though difficult to predict, and somewhere lost in this paradox is the importance of having peace of mind in order to enjoy a good night's sleep.

Peace of mind offers clarity. Yet there are so many barriers to peace of mind. You may have financial troubles and feel there's no way out. Your job may be stressful, and you can't leave it. Your marriage may be unsatisfying or disappointing. Perhaps you don't feel secure, you don't sleep well anymore, or you feel out of control. Perhaps your kids are getting into trouble, you feel that you've done something unforgivable, or a traumatic event in your life haunts you.

Naturally, it isn't fair that you suffer this way. Fortunately, there are many reasonable methods to help you attain peace of mind as long as you recognize, first and foremost, that you are in control of your own life. You ultimately make the decisions that will fix the problems and set you free. Yet you must make your voice heard. Declare yourself. Whether it's a spouse, your boss, or a coworker who is disturbing your peace of mind, make sure you explain calmly and confidently that things will have to change.

If it's a bad memory that keeps you awake, or if you've been victimized by someone who is no longer alive or is simply not accessible—a drunk driver, a lover who left you, a parent who abused you or neglected you—the solution is to get help. This situation may require an impartial third party: a kind, compassionate social worker; a psychologist; or a counselor who's been trained in short-term therapy (or longer, if necessary). It's covered by most insurance plans, and the results may surprise you. There's no need to be shy, stubborn, or old-fashioned about this; sometimes the best path to peace of mind is a simple adjustment of your point of view.

All in all, the three ingredients necessary for recovery described here—love, humor, and peace of mind—require a shift of perspective, a risky change, and a bit of courage. What better time to start than right now?

Fibromyalgia and Pregnancy

Even the healthiest woman can have a difficult time with pregnancy, whether it's morning sickness, insomnia, or simply fatigue. If you have fibromyalgia to begin with, however, it can be a double whammy. This doesn't mean you can't have a healthy, full-term pregnancy. At this point, there is little research to document the impact of fibromyalgia on pregnant women, although a 1997 Norwegian study found that pregnant women with fibromyalgia suffered more than usual while they were pregnant. The severity of symptoms continued until they were about three months past delivery. There was also a greater incidence of postpartum depression.

The babies, however, were born full term and healthy, so although the pregnancy may be more difficult for the woman with fibromyalgia, the outcome is the same as it is for any healthy woman.

On the other hand, some women with fibromyalgia have found that they actually feel better while pregnant, contradicting the findings of this study. Although they may have suffered from the initial fatigue and morning sickness, they began to feel better as they entered the following two trimesters. It is possible that this effect is due to the hormone relaxin, which increases tenfold when a woman is pregnant. Relaxin supplements have also been found to ease fibromyalgia symptoms.

Breastfeeding, however, can be even more difficult for the woman with fibromyalgia than it usually is, because of the chronic muscle pain. That is not to say it can't be done, but women with fibromyalgia need to keep the atmosphere stress-free and do everything possible to keep themselves comfortable if breastfeeding is important to them.

Certain tricks that work for other mothers are even more crucial if you have fibromyalgia. Find pillows to support the baby and yourself, or use a sling to hold the baby up. Lying on the bed with the baby at your side may also make feeding easier and can be restful. Stay away from the rest of your busy family or from distracting, chaotic places, and use your feeding time to relax and enjoy the baby.

There is no reason why women with fibromyalgia can't have the same satisfying experiences of pregnancy, childbirth, and breastfeeding that other women have.

Real-Life Stories of Recovery

Doreen was twenty-eight when she was rear-ended in a traffic accident on her way to work. The car was damaged enough that it had to be towed, but she showed no immediate injuries. She checked in at work, then went to the hospital for X-rays before going home. "I had no idea what was going to happen," she said.

Returning to work, she felt a little stiffness in her back and neck. Within two days, there was evidence of a mild traumatic brain injury, including headaches and dizziness, but she never anticipated any cognitive repercussions.

Doreen was married soon after the accident and continued a long commute to her teaching job. "All kinds of symptoms came up over the next couple of years," she said. "I found the commute to work very stressful."

At first, many symptoms seemed unrelated to the car accident. Doreen took some time off from her job and went to work at another school closer to her home while she visited one doctor after another. Finally, she found herself in the classroom completely bewildered. "I would walk into the classroom and not know where things were or what to do. I had to quit," she explained. Her therapist suspected Lyme disease, and she was tested for that. One physician prescribed pain medications and another prescribed Xanax and Paxil, then switched her to Celexa.

"I hated being on anything," she said. It was only when she found a rheumatologist who diagnosed fibromyalgia that she finally put all the pieces together. "He hooked me up with an awesome team of people, and he helped me get my sanity back." Doreen began cognitive rehabilitation, sessions with a therapist, physical therapy, yoga, Pilates, and regular exercise.

"Once I had the diagnosis, it put my mind at ease," she added. "Fibromyalgia is this invisible thing. I'd be at a party, and I'd just fall asleep, and then wake up in the morning and feel like a truck ran over me. People just don't get it."

"Diet was also a big part of this," she said. "I learned that I needed to eat every two to three hours to keep my metabolism where it should be. I realized that I was chemically sensitive, and I'm more sensitive to lights, noises, and smells." She started her own business with a wellness company that does marketing and referrals for safer products.

"Now I'm healthy, my husband's healthy, and my daughter's healthy, too. She'll be a year old soon, and that's the best medicine for me."

Doreen believes her recovery came about because her physician listened, validated what she said, and respected her wish to do things naturally. "He understood my need to do yoga and chiropractic," she added, "and I trusted him enough to do trigger point injections." Once she began to find the right path with treatment, she added, she was able to wean herself off all medications.

"I've taken the proactive stance. I was able to clear my mind and just heal," she said. "I was fortunate. My husband understood. My husband and family were behind me 100 percent."

In her quest for good health and balance, Doreen now realizes that she cannot eat too many carbohydrates. She takes vitamins regularly, plus supplements such as calcium. "I drink water all day and herbal tea at night. I've definitely noticed a huge difference.

"I am my own primary caregiver now. I advocate for myself. When times are stressful, I still feel pain in my neck and back, and my chiropractor is important to me. The symptoms don't bother me very long anymore."

Doreen hasn't gone back to teaching and admits that she misses it. "I'm not ready to step back into that place," she said. "Since the car accident, I'm just moving forward at my own pace. Fibromyalgia is still there, but it isn't keeping me from doing anything."

Sally, who holds down a high-powered administrative job, is forty-two and says she has had fibromyalgia for so long, it has just become part of her life.

"I have neck pain and hip pain—and suffered a neck injury previously," she explained. "Massage is really good, and yoga helps tremendously."

An old neck fracture that healed wrong triggers severe migraines, Sally explained, and this can sometimes be relieved by **pressure point therapy**.

Although coenzyme A has helped her, she recently stopped taking it and started with SAM-e, a product that is recommended for treating fibromyalgia and rheumatoid arthritis. "Coenzyme A is very expensive, and I thought if I tried something different, and more reasonable, it might be good." Not only did coenzyme A cost her $55 for sixty pills, but she felt it wasn't wise to take the same supplement all the time. Similarly, massage or pressure point therapy isn't always affordable, and after a job change she found it was no longer convenient to do yoga three times a week.

"When I did yoga, I didn't have pain or migraines," she said, "but that was when yoga classes were convenient and right at work. Naturopathic medicine also agrees with me more than traditional methods do, but it isn't covered by my insurance."

Sally, who has suffered from fibromyalgia for more than ten years, doesn't remember anything specific that triggered it, although she had a previous neck fracture and a few whiplash injuries.

"I was concerned at the time that I had Lyme, gout, or lupus," she said. "I also thought I had multiple sclerosis. If I get a migraine or the flu, it attacks my weak points. I can feel this grabbing hold of my muscles, can feel it moving from one side of my head to the other, to my joints and my hips. I have an intermittent focus problem, and it sometimes affects my speech, which affects my whole psyche."

If she remembers to do some exercise each day, she added, then she usually manages all right, "but if I don't do anything like stretching or exercise, I'm ready to fall on the floor by three P.M." Sally sits at a computer all day and said that the exercise is essential.

"The hardest part of fibromyalgia for me," she added, "is waking up, or sleeping through the night and not getting restful sleep."

During a difficult past year, she has started to take Cymbalta, which seems to be helping, and she sees a neurologist for the migraines. This doctor gave her Bextra, which tends to head off severe migraines. Changes in her diet included cutting out dairy and beginning to drink soy milk, adding **digestive enzymes** to her daily regimen, as well as **acidophilus** for healthy intestinal flora, and taking "enormous flaxseed pills with omega that are wonderful." Although she's had a difficult time recently, Sally said she was pleased with the recent changes she had made in supplements and medication; she understood her need for more exercise and stretching and felt that her overall condition was "on an upswing."

Susan, fifty-nine, is another woman who has experienced a range of fibromyalgia symptoms. She didn't have a car accident and still seems puzzled by what may have triggered this syndrome. "The pain just started one day out of the blue," she explained. "My internist ordered all sorts of tests, and I felt like I was losing my mind. I had three little girls and a big move coming up."

As she described her dilemma, she explained how the necessity for a cross-country move came when her three children were quite small. She knew she would be leaving family and friends who had been around her all her life. Her husband went ahead and found a new home and she was left with the kids, the packing, and all of the logistics of the move.

When she eventually settled into her new house, both of her parents became very ill, and her father-in-law actually died in her home.

"I knew that my body's response to these crises wasn't helping, but I couldn't control all these things," she said. Her internist pressed the trigger points and hinted at fibromyalgia. He prescribed Elavil and said she should get more exercise.

She was referred to a rheumatologist in order to screen out other immune system disorders, and she began treatment for fibromyalgia.

"There was no part of my body that didn't hurt or burn, like some deep, strange electrical thing," she explained. "The kids were between ten and twelve years old. I kept going and rarely got much rest during that first year when we had moved.

"My attitude before was that suffering was something you do in silence, and don't burden others with your problems," she said. "Now, I'm not afraid of speaking up. Now I talk. This is really happening, and we are going to do something about it."

Today, Susan goes to a massage therapist frequently, preferring a neuromuscular massage. She also participates in group yoga. "I'm better off as part of a group doing yoga," she said, "and I found someone who allows for all ranges of abilities. I also got a prescription for cyclobenzaprine, since interrupted sleep can bring on fibromyalgia, and menopause can interrupt sleep. I've learned that I always feel better if I've slept well."

Susan also visited the Center of Integrative Medicine in Boston and worked with a hypnotherapist in Andrew Weil's group there. "He took me through one session and taped it, and I listened to it every day for thirty days. Now I have that tape, plus another fibromyalgia CD to use." Hypnotherapy gave her relief from bouts of IBS, she said.

"I also drink ginger tea, take ginger supplements, eat ginger candy, and cook with ginger and turmeric," she said. "I take vitamins, calcium, vitamin C, glucosamine, and vitamin B-complex."

When her husband had a heart attack a few years ago, the couple eliminated junk food from their diets. "I lost twenty-five pounds over the last three years and eat more fruits and vegetables," she said.

Today, her symptoms are under control. "I remember being miserable in the early days," she said, "but I don't remember ever saying it. If you think you have fibromyalgia, first find a practitioner who will treat all of you. Try a mind-body approach, because medicine isn't an exact science, and I've found that natural alternatives work well, too. There's a role for medication in fibromyalgia, but you can't always run to the doctor for prescriptions."

Aimee, in her early twenties, also has a diagnosis of fibromyalgia and, like the other women mentioned in this chapter, got the diagnosis only after several years of searching for an answer to her problems.

"I had the idea that something was wrong with me," she said, "but nothing ever seemed to be found. I almost wanted someone to say lupus so that I could finally have an answer."

"I felt like I was crazy," she explained. "Nothing appeared to be wrong with me, but I felt lousy." Aimee suffered from bursitis in both hips and digestive problems. Finally, an optometrist mentioned that her eyes were dry, a symptom of arthritis, and when she mentioned this to her primary-care physician, he referred her to a rheumatologist. "This doctor put a name on what I had been feeling for two and a half years," she said. "It was the end of a long process."

Aimee recalled that she had contracted Lyme disease in college, which might have been the precursor of fibromyalgia. "I really noticed all these symptoms about six months after I started my first full-time job," she said. "When I started working, it really hit me. There's no down time as a high school French teacher. I start teaching at seven fifteen every morning, and I'm the worst morning person ever. I've had to make a lot of adjustments to keep up this pace."

Stress is also a precipitating factor that exacerbates her fibromyalgia symptoms. "I don't think I have a severe case of fibromyalgia," she said. "I always seem to be able to press on. I've made some lifestyle changes. Because I stand all day, I'm very careful about my shoes. I do yoga one or two times a week and exercise five times a week. It helps my energy level."

When she allows herself to become too tired and stressed, Aimee said, the pain in her hips and elbows worsens; she experiences overall fatigue and nausea. "If I get very tired, I have bad headaches," she added. "The symptoms seem to be cyclical. Everything descends on me for a while, and then it goes away."

To keep the symptoms at bay, Aimee has reduced sugar in her diet. "I am a vegetarian, and I maintain a very healthy diet," she said. "I was diagnosed with IBS before, and the medications didn't agree with me, but I found that drinking a lot of water helps."

Her biggest lifestyle change, however, revolves around sleep. "Sleep is superimportant to me," she said. "My room is dark and quiet, and everyone around me is quiet. Going to bed consistently early helps me get more quality sleep. When I'm not sleeping well, my fibromyalgia symptoms just get worse and worse."

If anything, the stories of these women illustrate even more clearly that fibromyalgia is a very individual disease. Onset and recovery never seem to be the same in two people. The variables of illness, accident, and trauma as triggering factors make fibromyalgia difficult to diagnose, and even when these women discovered the disease they actually had, the path to recovery was equally varied. The common denominator in every case was that these women had lost the delicate balance that had existed previously in their central nervous systems, and restoring this took a combination of medications, diet, exercise, supplements, and difficult lifestyle changes.

What these stories also prove is that there is a path to recovery, but it requires hard work on the part of both patient and physician. First, they must discover the precipitating factor for fibromyalgia and address that issue; then they must, through trial and error, find the therapies that are most beneficial and that will restore the patient to his or her previous good health.

If you have struggled with the symptoms of fibromyalgia for a long period of time, your recovery may be a bit slower. If you were diagnosed quickly after the onset of symptoms, you are more likely to face an easier recovery. You have to be the one to decide, with the input of your primary-care physician or specialist, which medications or treatments have the most impact on your symptoms. Your pain generators, the precipitating factor of your fibromyalgia, and your diet and exercise patterns are uniquely yours. Use the treatments described in the next chapter to create your own plan for wellness, adapt it as needed, and work with your caregivers to fine-tune the plan specifically for your needs.

11

Putting It All Together

Fibromyalgia is no longer a mystery syndrome. We know that it develops because of an ongoing injury to or imbalance inside the central nervous system. There is often a precipitating trauma or illness and frequently some kind of persistent pain generator. While treatment used to be primarily medication or giving up on an active lifestyle, we have described many popular holistic therapies that can be combined with conventional Western medicine. The emotional components of the syndrome—depression and insomnia, for example—do not mean that the fibromyalgia sufferer is weak or emotionally vulnerable. Something—heredity, an accident, an illness, or another trauma—predisposed you to fibromyalgia, but once the damage was done to the central nervous system, the symptoms and the pain continue and exacerbate your condition. As you pursue solutions, keep in mind that there is a way out of this dilemma.

Remember the following:

Fibromyalgia is a treatable imbalance of pain perception inside the central nervous system.

The sources of persistent pain must be uncovered and treated.

Fibromyalgia is either postinjury, illness-associated, or stress-associated.

Treatment options can range from pharmaceuticals, diet, and exercise to a whole range of alternative therapies.

You can find a way to live a full, productive life and keep all the symptoms under control.

There is a solution—and with the right tools you can find it!

The best fibromyalgia solution is a flexible one, adjusted according to your needs. Several paths have been suggested, based on the driving forces behind the symptoms. For convenience, the different types of fibromyalgia have been broken down into three categories: postinjury, illness-associated, and stress-associated. The purpose of subdividing fibromyalgia this way is to emphasize the aspects of care that may be necessary for the different sufferers. Thus, a person with post–Lyme disease fibromyalgia may have different needs than someone who has suffered an emotional shock or a neck injury.

In postinjury fibromyalgia, there may be less of a need for emotional or nutritional support than for an emphasis on physical modalities and pain management. In illness-associated fibromyalgia, there is a need to emphasize the body's natural defenses, neutraceutrical support and treatment of concurrent health issues. In stress-associated fibromyalgia, the main thrust of care should include mind-body medicine, relaxation techniques, and the treatment of underlying anxiety, depression, and insomnia.

Naturally, there are overlapping aspects when treating anyone who has fibromyalgia, but recognizing the three major subtypes brings us a step closer to individualized care.

As always, you should discuss all treatment options with your caregiver before you begin.

Patient 1: Postinjury Fibromyalgia

Our first patient is Jennifer, a busy thirty-year-old social worker who suffered a whiplash injury six months earlier. Her main symptom is pain, mostly around the neck and the lower back. The neck pain tends to radiate across her shoulders toward her upper arms. Not surprisingly, there is a great deal of stress in her life, both at work and at home. She spends her busy days helping others but has been unable to help herself, and she's getting worse.

She has fourteen symmetrical tender points above and below the waist; she is sleeping poorly, feels tired during the day, and has noticed frequent headaches. The pain has begun to interfere with her ability to concentrate at work. Jennifer is generally healthy and would like to avoid taking narcotic pain medication if possible.

The solution for Jennifer includes a combination of stress reduction, manual therapy, and prescription medication. Additional care for the ligamentous neck injury and intermittent migraine should be made available. The mainstay of pain relief, aside from medication, can include massage therapy, gentle chiropractic adjustments, trigger point injections, and **paracervical muscle relaxation**. MRI scanning of the head and the neck should be performed to rule out any insidious injury (such as a herniated disk) that can interfere with her recovery. A comprehensive physical exam and lab screening (outlined in chapter 7) will ensure that there is no other driving force behind the symptoms of Jennifer's fibromyalgia. Of greatest importance, Jennifer needs the support and understanding of thoughtful caregivers. If she is found to be healthy by her internist, it is quite reasonable for her follow-up care thereafter to be provided by a holistic practitioner. She may need to take a temporary break from the demands of work, and an emphasis on relaxation and light exercise will be key to her recovery.

The following program is a reasonable way to begin. For the most part, it emphasizes a mind-body approach to relaxation and a better environment for the healing of Jennifer's head and neck injury. The medications listed are entirely optional and flexible, and you may consider it a framework from which decisions can be made.

The use of safe, nonsedating medication is preferred, particularly for people who must continue to work. Stronger analgesics and muscle relaxants, if absolutely necessary, are best taken later in the day. Jennifer's treatment plan assumes that there is no herniated disk, spinal fracture, or unforeseen health problem. Since her fibromyalgia is probably being driven by a single traumatic event that's been perpetuated by daily chronic stress, this is what we propose (see the following table):

Treatment Plan

Activity/ Supplementation	Medication	Diet
MORNING		
Hot shower, gentle stretch/yoga	Nonsedating analgesic, topical NSAID	Coffee, juice, egg or cheese, whole-grain bread or muffin
Coenzyme Q10, antioxidant		
AFTERNOON		
Twenty-minute walk	Nonsedating analgesic, Pramipexole, Tiagabine	A well-rounded vegetarian meal that includes protein, vegetables, a serving of whole grain, fresh fruit, no caffeine

EVENING

Meditation, hot bath/Jacuzzi	Healthy protein, vegetables, serving of whole grain; no MSG, caffeine/cola, or aspartame

- There are several nonsedating analgesics on the market. A popular choice for fibromyalgia is the combination of tramadol and acetaminophen.

- Several topical nonsteroidal anti-inflammatory drugs are being tested in clinical trials. A good compounding pharmacy can prepare a topical mixture of naproxen, diclofenac, or ibuprofen for you. It can be applied to the tender spots around the neck or the lower back several times per day.

- Antioxidants such as vitamin C and E are available without a prescription. A popular brand is Juice Plus+.

- Trigger point injections can be performed at the paraspinal areas of muscle pain by an experienced physician on a monthly basis as needed (see chapter 9).

- Gentle manual therapy can begin once or twice weekly by a chiropractor, a massage therapist, or a physical therapist. After relief is found, treatment can be less frequent.

- If migraine headaches are an issue, topiramate, 50 mg, in the evening is often effective.

- Consider microcurrent treatments for tender points associated with cervical spine trauma.

So, what happened to Jennifer? First, she had a proper spinal and neurological investigation to exclude a cervical disk herniation, a cranial injury, or any other tangible source of head and neck pain. When it was determined that her symptoms were indeed derived from her whiplash injury six months earlier, she embarked on a program designed to restore a sense of comfort and well-being.

Unfortunately, a few legal issues surrounding the car accident needed to be better defined. Jennifer is not a vindictive person, but she is practical and understands that she has certain rights under the law. Since her health has been compromised, she needs reassurance that medical care will be available and her job will be preserved if time off work becomes necessary. This is one of the uglier aspects of postinjury care, where the powerful spheres of law and medicine merge, and it should not be overlooked. Suffice to say that Jennifer and her lawyer have agreed to be fair and honest as they forge ahead. Proper representation in this regard can remove a considerable amount of burden from Jennifer, who has no experience in such matters.

For better or worse, Jennifer's injury has been a wake-up call indicating that even before her car accident, she was set up to develop fibromyalgia. The constant stress in her life had a negative impact on her pain threshold, her immune system, her restorative sleep, and her ability to recover. With this new insight, she has promised herself that her life won't get out of control as it did in the past. She has readjusted her priorities at work and home and has removed some of the unbearable expectations she had previously placed on herself.

Her days have become more tolerable as a result, and the nagging symptoms of fibromyalgia are now manageable. She found considerable relief with a combination of massage and myofascial release techniques. Her physician targeted a few paracervical and mid-scapular trigger points and injected them with a combination of bupivacaine and Sarapin (a nontoxic derivative of the pitcher plant). She completed a tapering schedule of nonsedating analgesics and GABA-enhancing medication until she found relief.

It took nearly six months of treatment before Jennifer felt close to normal again, and her appreciation for the mind-body connection has been renewed. There are still a few nagging sore spots behind her neck, no doubt stemming from her ligament injury, but they never get out of hand. When Jennifer feels the knots in her muscles begin to tense up, she pays attention to these warning signs and finds help from her massage therapist and relaxation program.

Patient 2: Illness-Associated Fibromyalgia

Our next patient is Jean, a forty-year-old housewife who developed fibromyalgia during a lengthy search for the underlying cause of her chronic fatigue. Ultimately, she was found to have autoimmune thyroid disease, but even after a proper diagnosis, treatment, and a daily dose of thyroid replacement hormone, she continues to battle fatigue, insomnia, and muscle tenderness. She has a burning sensation in her skin that is most notable in the evening, at which time she tends to toss and turn in bed. She had always prided herself on being in excellent shape and on caring for her two young teens, but her illness has left her forty pounds heavier and quite uncomfortable.

If she were to continue in her present habits and lifestyle, Jean would most likely remain symptomatic. With patience, however, and the right combination of low-calorie diet, light aerobic exercise, and supportive medication, there's every reason to believe that she will make a complete recovery.

For Jean, the best approach to care is an integrative one. She needs the thoughtful monitoring of her medical condition by an internist with expertise in the field of endocrinology, and she also needs the ongoing care of a holistic practitioner well versed in the areas of diet, exercise, and wellness. Her prescribed routine is outlined in the following table

Treatment Plan

Activity/ Supplementation	Medication	Diet
MORNING		
Gentle stretch/yoga Coenzyme Q10, B-complex, ginkgo biloba, antioxidant	Thyroid replacement hormone, preferred analgesic, DHEA, Pregabalin	Coffee, juice, bran muffin, egg or cheese
AFTERNOON		
Twenty-minute walk, positive affirmations	Nonsedating analgesic	Sandwich on whole-grain bread, fresh fruit, yogurt
EVENING		
Group yoga	Preferred analgesic, Pregabalin, Cyclo-benzaprine, Ambien or Lunesta	Balanced vegetarian meal with protein, vegetables, and a serving of whole grain; no additives, caffeine, aspartame, or MSG

- The preferred analgesic may be tramadol or acetaminophen for mild pain or a nonsteroidal or COX-2 inhibitor if there is arthritis around the neck or the lower back. Hydrocodone may be appropriate on a limited basis for more severe pain.

- DHEA (dehydroepiandrosterone) can be helpful in this setting, although ask your doctor to check your baseline levels first.

- In clinical trials, the optimal dosage of pregabalin for fibromyalgia was 150 mg, three times per day, starting at 50 mg at bedtime and slowly increased as tolerated.

- Hypnotic sleeping agents should be taken on a night-by-night basis, only as needed and preferably not long term.

- A therapeutic massage given once or twice a week can make a world of difference.

- Aerobic exercise is a key to weight reduction and conditioning but should advance slowly according to tolerance.

Jean's improvement has been slow and steady. The changes in her body weight and energy were proportional to her gradual improvement in restorative sleep. As her muscle pain declined and the quality of her sleep improved, she noticed a measurable decline in her food cravings and a concomitant increase in energy. Ultimately, it took an entire year for Jean to achieve her optimal body weight, and she has faithfully adhered to the same program that fostered her recovery: proper diet, exercise, stress reduction, and sleep. She has tapered off all prescription medications, except for her thyroid supplement, and recognizes the warning signs of impending fibromyalgia activity that pop up from time to time.

Patient 3: Stress-Associated Fibromyalgia

Our third patient is Tina, a twenty-seven-year-old single professional woman with one year of escalating symptoms. Her diffuse pain has become excruciating despite the use of narcotic analgesics, and she fears the worst—loss of job security, loss of sanity, and loss of good health. Her primary-care physician has screened everything under the sun and has found nothing. Her chiropractor has performed X-rays of the neck and the back, which show only cervical straightening (a sign of muscle tension).

She has been calling in sick, has started smoking cigarettes, and has stayed in bed on most weekends. Her friends have become more distant. Her family is quite concerned. They are unaware of the secrets Tina has kept for more than ten years—that her older brother's friend had molested her when she was younger, and that Tina has spotted him in town recently. Although she cannot understand why these images have been interrupting her sleep or why they might be associated with her current symptoms, her physician has taken the time to explore these possibilities with her. Mindful of the stress and the anxiety she has faced lately, she has already embarked on a life-changing journey of stress reduction, light exercise, smoking cessation, and a pure vegetarian diet.

In Tina's case, there is no shortcut to wellness. The journey she must take is painstaking because her fibromyalgia has been stirred up by an upsetting dormant memory. Her health has been compromised as a result, and it will take great insight and acceptance to recover. With the right caregivers, including a thoughtful mental health worker well versed in the area of PTSD and a fibromyalgia expert who understands the subtle balance of pain, mood, and sleep, Tina can certainly recover. (A later note: she did.)

A healthier lifestyle that includes stress-reduction, removal of dietary neurotoxins, carefully tapering off narcotics, and a light exercise program has placed her on a more balanced path. Several prescription medications were necessary for a while, including an antidepressant that fostered a better mood and more restful sleep (see table below).

Treatment Plan

Activity/ Supplementation	Medication	Diet
MORNING		
Vitamin B-complex, ginkgo biloba, SAM-e	Duloxetine, preferred analgesic	Coffee, juice, egg or cheese, muffin
Light aerobic workout		
AFTERNOON		
Meditation, positive affirmations	Nonsedating analgesic	Fresh fruit, protein, vegetables, or salad, whole-grain bread; no dietary neurotoxins
EVENING		
Hot bath	Duloxetine, Tiagabine, Ambien or Lunesta, preferred analgesic	Well-balanced vegetarian dinner that includes protein, vegetables, and a serving of whole grain; no caffeine

- Duloxetine (Cymbalta) is an SNRI (see chapter 9) that should be started at the lowest possible dose to avoid side effects and gradually increased to a maximum daily dose of 120 mg.

- The preferred analgesic is always the safest nonsedating one; however, in Tina's case the first priority is to cautiously taper her off narcotic analgesics.

- SAM-e (S-adenosyl methionine) is a nonprescription supplement that has not held up very well in controlled studies of fibromyalgia, but if used judiciously, it can be a reasonable addition to an integrative program.

- In Tina's case, several aspects of desensitization will be most helpful. Options include one-on-one psychotherapy with a thoughtful social worker or psychologist with experience in PTSD (post-traumatic stress disorder), guided imagery, hypnosis, **eye movement desensitization and reprocessing (EMDR),** or virtual reality therapy when it becomes more widely available. If concurrent depression is an issue, particularly with a headache, a modern approach might include transcranial magnetic stimulation.

- A weekly or biweekly massage will be helpful to relax muscles and restore trust that she can be touched in a nonthreatening way.

Ultimately, Tina did well. Though she remains on an antidepressant once a day, she no longer requires a prescription for sleep or pain on a daily basis. Her job is secure, and her relationships are intact. She stopped smoking cigarettes early on and has faithfully continued her light aerobic workout every other day. After six months of weekly sessions with her psychotherapist, she has gained a greater awareness of the damage that was inflicted upon her. She will spend the rest of her life dealing with the harsh memories of her past—a wound that will no longer affect her health to the same degree. Her sense of security has been restored, and her feelings of optimism about the future have been renewed. She now volunteers once a month at a local women's shelter, where she provides comfort to people in need.

The cases outlined previously represent only a few examples of the many types of fibromyalgia seen in the community. Each case offers a glimpse at some of the available treatment options. No book can describe the hardships some people must face—their daily struggles and the cruel memories they silently endure. The association of tension and stress with the development of fibromyalgia cannot be overemphasized, and the mainstay of any fibromyalgia treatment program requires a soothing departure from relentless stress. Getting the tension out of your life is more important than anything. Listen to your body—it's trying to tell you this, and help is available. Read the entire contents of this book before rushing into one of the previous treatment plans, since a keen understanding of the mechanics involved in central sensitivity will undoubtedly offer you new insight, optimism, and hope. Good luck on your road to recovery!

APPENDIX A

Daily Coping Strategies

You can do lots of things to make your daily life more pleasant and less painful or stressful. We've suggested many of these within the text, but here's a list to refer back to, again and again:

1. Set your own pace for activities. Don't overextend yourself. You might be used to accomplishing a lot, but fibromyalgia changes things. Be ready to compromise.

2. Make time for yourself. This doesn't have to be a full hour set aside for yoga class or tai chi. It can be as simple as a fifteen-minute break for a cup of herbal tea while you watch the squirrels play outside. Let your mind go, and enjoy some peace and quiet.

3. If you are used to accomplishing a lot every day and are struggling with limited capabilities, set some realistic goals. Make a list, according to priorities, and check off the most important things first. If you don't finish, leave something for tomorrow, but you can at least look back at the list and feel that you did something concrete.

4. Avoid sitting for long periods of time. Get up and stretch. Move around. This applies to those of us who sit for long hours at a desk or computer or to anyone who is traveling. Stop

frequently and walk for a few minutes if you are driving, or, if you are on a plane, get up and stretch your legs.

5. Talk to other people who understand what you are going through. We've suggested some Web sites and chat rooms, but there are also support groups everywhere. Find other people who have fibromyalgia, and talk about what you are experiencing. Not only does this validate what you feel, but you might learn something useful from another person.

6. Avoid noxious smells, loud noises, and bright lights.

7. Keep your life as simple as possible, and eliminate any stressors that you can.

8. Don't assume that all the changes you must make are bad. Look for the positive impact these changes have on your life. In fact, look for everything positive. The better your outlook on life, the better you will feel.

9. If you have had to give up something you enjoy, think about what your skills and talents are. Could you share these with someone else? Finding a way to reinvent yourself—you were a great diver, but now you can be a great diving coach—may help you to find fulfillment in a changed life.

10. Take control of just one small aspect of your life, and excel at it. You may have been good at a lot of things, and because of fibromyalgia you had to let something slide. Now you can reclaim one thing and do it well. This will go a long way toward boosting your self-esteem and will make you feel better about your situation.

APPENDIX B

Managing Your Medical Information

Being diagnosed with fibromyalgia can be overwhelming. There is so much to learn and understand, and if your fibromyalgia results from an earlier trauma or illness, you will need to do a lot of soul-searching and work.

The diagnosis also means that you have a range of options to explore, from nutrition and exercise to medications and specific therapies. Although *Healing Fibromyalgia* has helped you to understand more about central sensitivity and how to treat certain symptoms, your own recovery is a unique process. Keeping track of office visits, medications, alternative therapies, and dietary changes can make your life simpler to navigate later on.

You can do this in lots of ways, and it doesn't have to be too technical. Just pick out a notebook that is a comfortable size for you, something easy to write in. Some people may want to carry it in a briefcase or a purse to and from work and office visits, or it might end up on your bedside table where you can jot down notes at the end of the day. Whatever works for you is fine.

Begin at the very beginning. When did you first notice the symptoms of fibromyalgia? Perhaps it was six months after that nasty car accident. Maybe you had severe muscular pain, unrelated to any physical trauma, but it seemed to start sometime after the death of a favorite relative or a close friend. Maybe you can't even make this kind of connection, but you know it was in the middle of the winter and you suddenly discovered that you were too tired and sore to sweep an inch of snow off the sidewalk.

Go back to that moment, and record it in your journal. You don't have to understand exactly what the connections might be to previous traumas or accidents, but simply journaling may bring you to some realization.

Now, go back to this journal on a regular basis. Record your first visit to the physician to talk about these symptoms. What were his or her recommendations? Did the physician give you any prescriptions? Did he or she have any other treatment ideas?

If you were lucky enough to get an accurate diagnosis early on, begin some research on your own. You want to understand exactly what you are dealing with. Keep track of your symptoms, related or not. You can decide later (or let your doctor decide) whether the tingling in your fingers has something to do with fibromyalgia.

Perhaps your physician begins by prescribing a low dose of an antidepressant such as Prozac, for depression. You can read the flyers that accompany prescriptions from the pharmacy, but it might be more useful just to keep track of how you feel.

For instance:

Day 1 on Prozac—No difference.

Day 2—No difference.

Day 3—No difference.

Day 4—Perhaps it's positive thinking on my part, but things seem better.

Day 5—I think I'm feeling better.

Day 6—I feel better and have more energy.

Day 7—Now I know I feel better, but I'm jittery. Is it the medicine?

You can follow a similar pattern with any medication that you try. Maybe the muscle relaxant helps you to achieve more restful sleep and reduces muscle spasms but leaves you feeling groggy in the morning. Keep track of the extent of your grogginess each day, and maybe you'll suddenly discover that you have adjusted to this medication. Perhaps it is helping and not really hindering, and it might be a good idea to continue taking it to reduce your symptoms for the short term.

Keep track of what happens during office visits. If you've asked questions and haven't gotten good answers, jot down a note to ask that question again. Keep a log of phone calls to the physician's office. If too many things happen at once, then it becomes difficult to sort out what Prozac did compared to what the muscle relaxant did.

This becomes really important when you try to modify your diet. Perhaps you have been plagued by headaches for months. You cut out aspartame, and the headaches stop for three weeks and start again. Was it the aspartame or has something else changed? If you can look back in your journal and note that you also stopped drinking coffee or wine, you have a better chance of coming to the correct conclusion.

Make the journal a useful tool in your quest for good health. Don't become obsessed with keeping track of every detail. In other words, don't dwell on every symptom, ache, and pain, but be aware of what medications you take, what foods you eat, how you feel the day after tai chi, and what your spirits are like.

A journal, in and of itself, can be therapeutic. As you jot down thoughts about how a physician treated you or how your spouse reacted when you told him or her about tender points, more might be revealed than you expect. Two weeks later, you may look back and realize that you were upset by what happened, but you didn't even acknowledge it to yourself. Lots of feelings get sorted out in the writing process, and this can be a valuable tool as you continue on your journey to wellness.

APPENDIX C

Navigating the Insurance Hurdles

The business of health insurance has changed dramatically in the last ten years. Physicians who used to be paid more for providing more services now have to be wary of offering more than the insurance company is willing to reimburse. In addition, many of the strategies or treatments that are suggested for fibromyalgia may not even be covered by some companies.

If you have fibromyalgia, take a close look at your insurance policy. What is covered, and what isn't, will be spelled out. Typically, visits to your physician require your co-pay and aren't restricted. Visits to a specialist probably require a referral, and there may be a maximum number of visits allowed during a certain time period.

Perhaps your doctor will refer you to a rheumatologist or may recommend physical therapy or chiropractic and massage, plus psychological counseling for some unresolved emotional issues that might have contributed to the onset of fibromyalgia. What you don't need right now is to build up a pile of medical bills that you can't afford to pay, so it is important to be clear about what kind of services are covered, and which aren't.

If you are in doubt, check with your insurance carrier. Be sure that if your physician recommends another kind of treatment, you get a referral before the starting date of the new services.

Many insurance plans require a co-pay for each office visit, although lab work and X-rays might be covered entirely. Physical therapy, chiropractic, and counseling are also usually covered, but something like massage usually isn't. You'll have to decide how important a massage or a yoga class is and whether the cost is equivalent to the benefit that you receive.

This is another situation where your journal might be useful. You can document office visits and alternative therapies, co-pays, and other expenses, and be prepared to present such information to your insurance company.

Just because you need it, and it's good for you, doesn't mean your insurance company will pay for it. These firms tend to stay on the side of conventional Western medicine, despite evidence that supports alternative treatments. Be prepared to pick up the tab on some things that might be important to you but that insurance won't cover.

If you find that you are unable to keep up with your work and must take an extended leave of absence or quit, there are resources to help you pay the resulting living and medical expenses. Perhaps you need to find an attorney to be your advocate in this situation, or, if you have the time and energy, investigate it yourself.

Fibromyalgia is an accepted diagnosis for disability, and you can qualify for this help if necessary.

APPENDIX D

Creating the Optimal
Work Environment

Getting through the week can be hard enough, but when you've got fibromyalgia, it's even tougher. Work environments can make symptoms worse or, at best, hinder your recovery. Figure out what you need to do to make your work situation as comfortable and pleasant as possible.

If you must sit at a desk all day, be diligent about getting up every fifteen or twenty minutes and moving around. Long-term sitting can lead to stiffness that exacerbates fibromyalgia symptoms. If you work at a computer, be sure that you have an ergonomic chair and keyboard. Whatever you can do to minimize stress and strain will benefit you in the long run.

Different things can impact fibromyalgia sufferers in a variety of ways. Blinking fluorescent lights might bring on a headache, or loud noises and noxious smells might trigger your symptoms. It is reasonable to ask your employer to reduce such harmful stimuli as much as possible. Perhaps you are seated by a drafty window. Bring a shawl or a small blanket to throw over your shoulders, or ask for a space heater to keep yourself comfortable. It is to everyone's advantage to keep you comfortable and working at maximum productivity.

If you must stand for long periods or perform repetitive tasks, such as on an assembly line, ask for any modifications that will help you to do a better job and will keep you from being too uncomfortable. This might be as simple as the option of sitting on a stool for short periods or alternating repetitive tasks with another job that isn't as stressful.

Do you have a clear, unobstructed path to the restroom and the freedom to take restroom breaks frequently? If you're the only one on the switchboard for four hours at a time, it's not unreasonable to ask that someone else be ready to take over for five minutes here and there to give you a much-needed break.

It isn't only the unskilled worker who suffers from workplace stress and injury or who puts up with conditions that may make fibromyalgia worse. Anyone can be in a drafty office, have an uncomfortable chair, be expected to lift heavy boxes of papers, and so on. If you had a broken bone or some other easily identified injury, people would go out of their way to help you. You wouldn't be expected to spring up the stairs on your crutches and carry a heavy load back down. It's no different with fibromyalgia; although no one can see your discomfort, it's still there. It's up to you to protect your health and take whatever precautions are necessary.

If you don't work outside the home, you should nevertheless consider what you do as "your work." Pace yourself, take on reasonable tasks, ask for help when you need it, and avoid unnecessary stress or injury. Many injuries happen in the home. It's frustrating to want to hang a new picture on the wall or move the refrigerator six inches to the left or the couch across the room, yet not be able to do it; however, tackling too many physical tasks when you have fibromyalgia will leave you in worse shape than before. Think twice before you start moving the furniture around or even before you clean out the kitchen pantry. How much can you reasonably handle in a day? Will the sight of all your dishes and pans stacked up on the table overwhelm you by the next day? Have realistic expectations. Just like overdoing exercise, overdoing household chores can set you back, and it isn't worth it.

Remember that lots of normal people with an abundance of energy can't finish their "to do" list every day. Take comfort in the fact that whatever you have done, it is enough. The goal in life is not to see how much you can accomplish in how little time, but to live each day to the fullest.

The Disability Issue

The Social Security Administration defines disability as "an inability to perform substantial gainful activity because of a medically determinable physical or mental impairment which can be expected to last for a continuous period of not less than 12 months." From a medical-legal standpoint, the problem of fibromyalgia becomes murky; although the symptoms of fibromyalgia generally do not resolve within twelve months, the complaints are largely subjective in nature, and there may be a job description (other than yours) that you are capable of performing. For this reason, a designation of long-term disability in fibromyalgia is difficult to attain.

As far as temporary disability, there are laws designed to protect employees who are unable to function for a defined period of time. Maternity leave is commonplace, and during the months out of work, one's motivation rarely comes into question. A fractured pelvis suffered during a ski vacation is understood, after which there may be "welcome back" balloons and a cake. What about fibromyalgia, though? When is it reasonable to request a period of temporary disability?

The answer varies depending upon the severity of symptoms, the physical and emotional demands of work, and the options for alternative employment. Some people lack the language or the technical skills to perform sedentary level work; others may consider themselves unable to work under any circumstances. And while this may be true for certain individuals, there are also examples of people with fibromyalgia who simply hate their jobs and attempt to get permanent total disability. The resulting impasse between employers and insurers on one side and patients (and their physician advocates) on the other needs to be further clarified for the benefit of everyone involved.

The process generally begins when an employee with fibromyalgia believes he or she can no longer function well enough to meet the demands of work. If desired, this individual may discuss the dilemma with his or her boss or a representative from the human resources department. This discussion may include options to adjust his or her work schedule or the particular requirements of the job. Depending on the situation, the employee may wish to give fair notice that he or she requires a period of time off work for medical reasons. Upon doing so, the employee can contact the Social Security Administration or the State Department of Disability Services and sign a waiver that gives it permission to request his or her medical records.

Interestingly, your doctor does not have the authority to designate you disabled or not, although he or she may serve as your advocate and may support your application. The state makes the ultimate decision that determines you to be disabled and for how long. Furthermore, the details of your disability insurance plan may dictate whether you're entitled to financial compensation during your time out of work.

In many cases, the medical record, despite a physician's documented empathy and advocacy of a patient's request for disability, will not sufficiently support an application for long-term disability. Too often, there is a lack of objective data needed to confirm the diagnosis: for example, the absence of exclusion of other causes of symptoms and insufficient details of the tender points on physical examination. Thus, the subjective complaint of pain, while unfortunate, does not necessarily incapacitate an employee from performing

U.S. Department of Labor
Work Classifications

The U.S. Department of Labor classifies five degrees of work in terms of the strength and the endurance required as follows:

1. *Sedentary Level Work*: Lifting 10 pounds maximum and occasionally lifting and/or carrying such articles as dockets, ledgers, and small tools. Although a sedentary job is defined as one that involves sitting, a certain amount of walking and standing is often necessary in carrying out job duties. Jobs are sedentary if walking and standing are required only occasionally and other sedentary criteria are met.

2. *Light Level Work*: Lifting 20 pounds maximum, with frequent lifting and/or carrying of objects weighing up to 10 pounds. Even though the weight lifted may be only a negligible amount, a job is in this category when it involves sitting most of the time with a degree of pushing and pulling of arm and/or leg controls, or when it requires walking or standing to a significant degree.

3. *Medium Level Work*: Lifting 50 pounds maximum, with frequent lifting and/or carrying of objects weighing up to 25 pounds.

4. *Heavy Level Work*: Lifting 100 pounds maximum, with frequent lifting and/or carrying of objects weighing up to 50 pounds.

5. *Very Heavy Level Work*: Lifting objects in excess of 100 pounds, with frequent lifting and/or carrying of objects weighing 50 pounds or more.

---

work. For example, if a person with fibromyalgia complains that his or her symptoms have become too unbearable to reach overhead and stack shelves or stand up for more than a few hours a day, this individual may be cleared for a more sedentary job.

From an employer's standpoint, your job description may simply require an adjustment in the number of work hours or in the physical demands in order to keep you more comfortable at work. Placing limitations within the boundaries of sedentary level work can offer a reasonable compromise, although there isn't always agreement about this. Such adjustments are more likely possible in larger corporations in which lateral movement can occur between different offices; however, smaller businesses have less opportunity for job flexibility. A self-employed person with fibromyalgia may have even less flexibility to adjust his or her schedule or job demands.

If there is a discrepancy between a fibromyalgia sufferer's ability to work and the job demands of his or her employer, a third party such as an independent medical evaluator (IME) sometimes steps in to render an impartial opinion. If there is still disagreement, an individual can seek legal advice from an attorney, and a hearing can be requested. In most cases, a reasonable compromise is found whereby a person receives a period of temporary disability before returning to work at a more realistic level of functioning.

Beyond the frustration of not being able to meet the physical demands of a job, a frequent obstacle to employment for people with fibromyalgia may be the emotional stress of the workplace. Job stress can be pernicious indeed and can easily perpetuate the symptoms of fibromyalgia in susceptible individuals. An unhealthy work environment may include a barrage of duties, a relentlessly hectic pace, exposure to personal humiliation such as sexual harassment, or simply job dissatisfaction. Between Monday and Friday, if you spend the majority of your waking hours at work and your job is not rewarding on some level, the specter of fibromyalgia becomes even more unbearable. Yet if you request time off work because of a flare-up of fibromyalgia, the goal of obtaining long-term disability may not be your best option. Your ultimate goal should always be a healthy recovery, even if you've been symptomatic for years. You will usually be able to return to a comfortably productive lifestyle, although you may first need to undergo a period of temporary disability.

Short-term disability generally lasts between three and six months, during which time an employer may continue to pay your normal salary, usually before long-term disability insurance kicks in. During this important time when you're out of work, a recovery can reasonably be expected to occur. Initially, your time off work should emphasize rest and restorative sleep, pain relief, and relaxation. You would follow this weeks later with a gradual increase in light aerobic activity and mind-body work such as therapeutic massage. When you discuss your eventual return with the human resources department or directly with your employer, you should negotiate a realistic adjustment of the workload expected of you. If you are self-employed, you may want to return to work part time at first.

Ultimately, if you attempt to return to work without following the aforementioned advice, you will likely relapse. Don't let this happen. If you feel pressured to perform at an unrealistic level, consider your options and get assistance. In a perpetually unforgiving work environment, your best choice may be to walk away and find different employment. Otherwise, seek legal advice. Fortunately, the majority of people with fibromyalgia remain gainfully employed despite their limitations; they make adjustments at work and home while avoiding the aggravating stressors that invariably come along. Most jobs offer full benefits for an abbreviated thirty-two-hour workweek, and you'd be surprised to learn how many employers are willing to make adjustments for their valuable employees with fibromyalgia.

RESOURCES

Organizations

The American Fibromyalgia Syndrome Association
6380 E. Tanque Verde, Suite D
Tucson, AZ 85715
520-733-1570
www.afsafund.org

   This is the only charitable organization devoted solely to funding research on fibromyalgia and chronic fatigue. Even though you may not be a physician involved in research, there are a wealth of articles on current research projects, a way to make donations to research, and sections on patient advocacy.

Fibrohugs.com
167 Scarth Street N.
Regina, SK
Canada S4R 2Z4
306-569-2077
www.fibrohugs.com

   This site features message forums, chat rooms, and a newsletter. Fibromyalgia is a very individual disease, so remember that what works for someone else will not necessarily work for you. It can ease your burden, however, if you keep in mind that millions of people are out there with the same symptoms as you. Use the chat rooms and the message forums to communicate with others, particularly if you don't have the option of attending a support group. Be a skeptic about any advice you get online, though; it might be nice to have online friends who understand your predicament, but they can't replace a good physician or caregiver who knows you personally and can see your recovery.

Fibromyalgia Support Network
c/o Global Healing Center
2040 North Loop West, Suite 108
Houston, TX 77018
www.fibromyalgia-support.org

This site has interesting material on fibromyalgia symptoms, coping techniques, and more. The site primarily promotes the network's own product, which is a blend of herbs and glyconutrients.

Fibromyalgia Network (quarterly journal)
P.O. Box 31750
Tucson, AZ 85751
800-853-2929
www.fmnet.news.com

This site contains a useful section on "Coping Tips." It also has a Web Store from which you can order specific materials. This might be useful if you have a question or an issue that hasn't been resolved through other channels, and you want a particular pamphlet. If you are a subscriber, the site also offers referrals to physicians. Again, getting another person who shares your experiences to recommend a physician might work just as well.

Fibromyalgia Frontiers Journal
National Fibromyalgia Partnership, Inc.
140 Zinn Way, P.O. Box 160
Linden, VA 22642-5609
866-725-4404
www.fmpartnership.org

This nonprofit organization offers a wide variety of free information on its Web site, or you can write for the NFP brochure and catalog by sending a self-addressed stamped envelope to the above address. Membership in this organization is $25 a year and includes its newsletter.

Fibromyalgia Association UK
P.O. Box 206
Stourbridge DY9 8YL
United Kingdom
www.fibromyalgia-associationuk.org

This is a nonprofit organization dedicated to education. It offers information about support groups in the United Kingdom, Ireland, and Channel Isles, publishes an online magazine called *FaMily*, and provides links to approved products and services. The focus of the educational materials is on current research and self-management.

The Fibromyalgia Connection
The Fibromyalgia Association of Houston
P.O. Box 2174
Bellaire, TX 77402
713-664-0180
www.fmah.org

This organization publishes a newsletter three times a year. There are also links to research sites, news of Texas-based support groups and forums, and articles on new studies.

National Fibromyalgia Association
220 N. Glassel Street, Suite A
Orange, CA 92865
714-921-0150
www.fmaware.org

This site includes an interesting article on men and fibromyalgia: "It's a Guy Thing: Men with Fibromyalgia." It also publishes *Fibromyalgia Aware* magazine and the quarterly report *Metamorphosis*, as well as provides information on clinical trials, support group directories, and links to advertisers.

FibroManage.com

This is a natural wellness site that sells items for fibromyalgia, such as aromatherapy and Ayurvedic medicine products and homeopathy and nutritional supplements. Like many other sites that are recommended here, however, it might be useful for learning about various treatment options, nutrition, supplements, and therapeutic tools. It's a good idea to discuss any ideas with your physician before you try something new.

National Institute of Arthritis, Musculoskeletal and Skin Diseases
P.O. Box AMS
9000 Rockville Pike
Bethesda, MD 20891

301-495-4484 or 877-22-NIAMS (toll free)
www.niams.nih.gov

This organization offers a free packet of fibromyalgia information and the American College of Rheumatology's fact sheet.

Oregon Fibromyalgia Foundation
120 NW 9th Avenue, Suite 216
Portland, OR 97205
503-228-3217
www.myalgia.com

This organization is a nonprofit with no commercial endorsements, but it is unable to answer individual questions.

Health Points is the newsletter of To Your Health (TYH), which is based in Fountain Hills near Phoenix, Arizona. This organization has labs and a research staff for its supplements and vitamins. Subscribe to the newsletter by calling 800-801-1406. The cost of $20 to join is applied to your first order.

Fibromyalgia Association Created for Education and Self-Help (FACES)
4281 W. 76th Street, Suite 501
P.O. Box 528504
Chicago, IL 60652
773-936-4138
www.fibrocop.org

This site provides education and self-help advice. It's a good source of information about what's happening in research but is strictly supplemental—not the place to go for everything you need to know.

FM/CFS Canada
99 Fifth Avenue, Suite 412
Ottawa, ON K1S 5P5
Canada
877-437-4673
www.fm-cfs.ca

This site with offers recent research articles, a section on legal research, book selections, videos, and a directory of support groups.

Resources for Disability Issues

fmnetnews.com—click on "Advocacy"

ssa.gov.disability (Social Security online)

ICDRI—International Center for Disability Resources on the Internet

Other suggestions: Web sites put up by attorneys might give you ideas about filing for disability, but this isn't necessarily the best way to find the right attorney, any more than it is a good way to find a doctor.

Sources for Pain Management

www.painrelieffoundation.org

www.painreliefnetwork.org

www.headaches.org

Sources for Irritable Bowel Syndrome

www.ibsgroup.org

www.aboutibs.org

Medical Journals

Journal of Musculoskeletal Pain and the *Journal of Chronic Fatigue*
Order from Medical Press, 800-429-6784 or visit www.HaworthPress.com
   In Volume 11, Number 4 (2003), there is a particularly good article on fibromyalgia titled "The Canadian Consensus Report." The article is written in an easy-to-understand fashion and will help you learn more clinical information about the syndrome.

Journal of Musculoskeletal Medicine
Cliggot Publishing Company
P.O. Box 4010
Greenwich, CT 06830

Web Sites

www.psych.org (American Psychiatric Association)

www.nmha.org (National Mental Health Association)

www.ncptsd.org/facts (National Center for Post-Traumatic Stress Disorder)

http://webmd.com/hw/health_guide (exercise and fibromyalgia)

www.spine.org

www.ninds.nih.gov/disorders/whiplash

www.nih.gov/medlineplus

www.familydoctor.org

www.fibromyalgia-symptoms.org/fibromyalgia/treatments

www.neurologychannel.com/fibromyalgia/treatments

www.uwnews.org

www.healthfinder.gov.news

www.arthritis.org

www.ichelp.org (interstitial cystitis)

www.kidney.niddk.nih.gov (interstitial cystitis)

www.mayoclinic.com

http://science-education.nih.gov

www.sleepnet.com

www.smilingfibros.net

www.members.fortunecity.com

www.cdc.gov

www.rheumatology.org

www.nfra.net (National Fibromyalgia Research Association)

www.fmscommunity.org

www.fmaware.org

www.chronicfatigue.about.com

www.myopain.org

fibrobetsy@rcn.com

GLOSSARY

acetylcholine   A neurotransmitter that regulates cardiovascular tone and daytime alertness.

acidophilus   Naturally occurring bacteria that assist digestion.

acupuncture points   Areas of the body into which the insertion of small needles may stimulate the body's natural energy and healing mechanisms.

adenosine   A peptide.

allodynea   A term that means feeling pain everywhere.

allopathic   A term for traditional Western medicine; it includes preventive measures, health screening, prescription medications, and surgery.

alpha-2 delta receptor blockers   Agents that affect voltage-regulated calcium channels in the central nervous system.

alpha waves   These are faster brain waves that intrude upon the slower waves of restful sleep.

amino acids   The smallest building blocks of proteins.

amitryptyline   The generic name of a tricyclic antidepressant that is marketed under the brand name Elavil.

amygdala   The brain's primitive emotional center.

amyloidosis   The accumulation of an insoluble protein fiber around the nerves.

aspartate   An essential amino acid; also, a neurotransmitter involved in long-term potentiation.

bone scanning   A diagnostic tool that is used to detect areas of increased or decreased bone mass.

bruxism   The act of grinding one's teeth while asleep.

buccinator   The muscles involved in chewing that are prone to myofascial pain and shortening.

bupivacaine   A painkiller or a type of anesthesia.

central sensitivity   An imbalance of either neurotransmitters or excitatory amino acids in the central nervous system that causes a heightened awareness of external stimuli.

cerebellar tonsils   The lowest part of the brain; it is vulnerable to compression in people who have Arnold-Chiari malformation.

cerebrospinal fluid   A clear substance that flows over the surface of the brain, provides nourishment, and cushions the brain against a sudden jarring or minor injury.

cervical spondylosis   Degenerative changes of the cervical spine that may contribute to pain and muscle spasm.

circadian rhythm   The day-night balance within the body of waking and sleeping.

coenzyme Q10 supplement   A supplement with antioxidant effects; it helps in the production of energy.

complex regional pain syndrome   See RSD.

corticotropin-releasing hormone (CRH)   A hormone released by the hypothalamus, which activates the pituitary gland to release ACTH (adrenocorticotropic hormone).

cortisol   A hormone produced by the adrenal gland in response to stress; it helps to maintain electrolyte balance and vascular tone.

cryoanalgesia   The application of a freezing substance to tissue to block painful nerve impulses.

cyclobenzaprine   The generic name of a tricyclic antidepressant that is marketed under the brand name Flexeril.

cytokines   Inflammatory mediators such as TNF-alpha and interleukin-1; they contribute to the flulike aching and the fatigue of fibromyalgia and also amplify the pain messages received by the brain.

dextromethorphan   A narcotic that is used in cough medicines.

digestive enzymes   Enzymes that are naturally produced by the body and are also sold as supplements; they help break down foods into nutrients the body can use.

dopamine   A key inhibitory neurotransmitter that regulates muscle control, sleep, and pain.

dopaminergic agents   Agents that are used to increase dopamine output.

dorsal horn   The posterior column of the spinal cord that regulates sensory information.

duloxetine   The generic name of a dual uptake inhibitor (SNRI) that is marketed under the brand name Cymbalta.

dysautonomia   The intermittent weakness and dizziness found in up to 30 percent of people with fibromyalgia.

electroencephalogram (EEG)   A device that measures brain wave patterns.

endorphins   The body's natural painkillers.

eszopiclone   The generic name of a sleep agent that is marketed under the brand name Lunesta.

eye movement desensitization and reprocessing (EMDR)   A technique used in conjunction with psychotherapy to help people deal with post-traumatic stress.

fibromyalgia   A syndrome of widespread pain and fatigue.

fish oil   Oil from fatty species of fish that contains omega-3 EPA and DHA, essential fatty acids that are not produced by the body but are essential to cardiovascular health and normal brain development.

fluoxetine   The generic name of a selective serotonin reuptake inhibitor marketed under the brand name Prozac.

foramen magnum   The canal through which the spinal cord descends.

frontal cortex   The part of the brain that regulates behavior.

gamma-amino-butyric acid (GABA)   An inhibitory neurotransmitter produced in the ventrolateral preoptic area, the sleep center of the brain.

ganalin   A peptide released in the sleep center of the brain.

glial cell   A cell that is derived from immune cell lineage; it is part of the supporting architecture of the central nervous system and can produce inflammatory cytokines.

glutamate   An essential amino acid; it is also a neurotransmitter involved in long-term potentiation.

Grave's disease   A common type of hyperthyroidism, in which the thyroid gland produces too much thyroid hormone.

Hashimoto's thyroiditis   Autoimmune thyroiditis; an inflammation of the thyroid gland in which the body's autoimmune response sends cells to attack the thyroid gland. This causes part or all of the gland to lose function and ultimately results in hypothyroidism, an inability to produce enough thyroid hormone.

hatha yoga   A meditative, low-impact type of exercise that features stretching, strength, and deep breathing.

hippocampus   The sensitive area of the brain in which memory is stored; it is vulnerable to trauma and chronic stress.

histamine   A compound that promotes allergic reactions, inflammation, and pain; it also helps to keep you alert and awake.

hormone   A substance released into the bloodstream from a gland or an organ to affect activity at another bodily site.

hyperalgesia   Abnormally high sensitivity to pain.

hypersomnia   Excessive daytime sleepiness.

hypnic myoclonia   Sudden muscle contractions during stage 1 sleep.

hypothalamic-pituitary-adrenal axis (HPA axis)   A major part of the neuro-endocrine system that controls reactions to stress and regulates various body processes including the immune system.

hypothalamus   The master thermostat of the brain; it regulates endocrine function.

integrative medicine   The combination of standard and holistic medicines.

interleukin-1   An inflammatory mediator or cytokine; it produces fever and inflammation.

interleukin-6   An immune-mediated messenger that promotes inflammation, pain, and fatigue.

interleukin-10   A naturally occurring anti-inflammatory cytokine.

interstitial cystitis   An irritation or an imbalance of the bladder that produces painful urination.

ions   An atom or a group of atoms that produces a net electrical charge.

ketamine   An NMDA inhibitor that is used as an anesthetic.

learned behavior   Behavior that is modified by previous experience or observation.

lecithin   A waxy phospholipid that has emulsifying and antioxidant properties; it supports the myelin sheath of nerves.

lidocaine   A local anesthetic.

limbic system   The primitive part of the brain that regulates feelings of suffering and stress.

lipids   Small fatty building blocks that make up certain neurotransmitters.

locus ceruleus-norepinephrine center   The area of the brain that maintains wakefulness.

long-term potentiation (LTP)   The accumulation of messages required for complex thinking or activity.

Lyme disease   A spirochetal infection acquired from a deer tick bite; it is most common in the northeastern United States.

maladaptive pain behavior   Counterproductive behavior that arises in response to pain.

malocclusion   Crowded or misaligned teeth.

masseter   The muscle of mastication, or chewing.

mechanical pain   Pain that usually arises after a trauma, although it can also be structural, developmental, postural, or degenerative in nature.

memantine   The generic name of an NMDA receptor antagonist that is marketed under the brand name Namenda.

membrane-stabilizing medication   A medication that normalizes the effects of excitatory neurotransmitters.

milnacipran   The generic name of a dual uptake inhibitor (SNRI) that is marketed under the brand name Ixel.

monosodium glutamate (MSG)   A food additive that may augment the excitatory effects of glutamate.

multiple sleep latency test   A sleep test that is given the day after a person undergoes a polysomnography to determine the extent of sleep deprivation.

myofascial pain   A regional muscular pain syndrome, whether post-trauma or postural, that arises due to the shortening or tension of muscle fibers.

narcolepsy   A sleep disorder associated with unpredictable paroxysms of deep sleep.

nerve compression   When shortened muscles (as in myofascial pain) or other body parts (ligaments, tendons) compress certain nerves and cause pain, numbness, and tingling in a region of the body beyond the compression.

nerve growth factor   A substance that stimulates growth and differentiation of the sympathetic and sensory nerves; it is found in abnormally high levels in fibromyalgia sufferers.

neurons   The cells of the nervous system that carry messages.

neurotransmitters   Peptides or hormones that affect local or distant nerve function.

N-methyl-D-aspartate (NMDA)   A substance that contributes to the amplification of pain and the "wind-up" effect seen in fibromyalgia.

nonmechanical pain   Pain resulting from an abnormal sensation, an inflammation, or a disease.

nonsteroidal anti-inflammatory drugs (NSAIDs)   Drugs that block certain enzymes and reduce prostaglandins throughout the body. This reduces inflammation, pain, and fever.

norepinephrine   One of the stress hormones; it constricts blood vessels, affects the pulse and blood pressure, and facilitates focus and attention.

nortriptyline   The generic name of a tricyclic antidepressant that is marketed under the brand name Pamelor.

orexin   A substance released in the HPA axis to regulate the brain's arousal center.

pain generator   An unyielding source of chronic pain.

paracervical muscle relaxation   A type of relaxation therapy that provides relief from tension headaches and neck pain.

paroxetine   The generic name of a selective serotonin reuptake inhibitor (SSRI) marketed under the brand name Paxil; an antidepressant.

pelvic obliquity   A tilting of the pelvis to one side.

Pilates   A series of exercises that focuses on improving flexibility and strength.

polymyalgia rheumatica (PMR)   An inflammatory disorder causing widespread muscle aches and stiffness.

polysomnography   A sleep study that determines types of sleep disorders.

positive thinking   Using positive images and thoughts to eradicate the negative ones that may impinge upon a healthy lifestyle.

post-traumatic stress disorder (PTSD)   Stress, anxiety, and difficulty in coping that originates from a prior trauma, either physical or emotional.

prednisone   A corticosteroid that is used to treat arthritis; it helps to reduce swelling and changes the way the immune system works.

pregabalin   The generic name of an alpha-2 delta receptor blocker that is marketed under the brand name Lyrica. It is used primarily to treat nerve pain.

pressure point therapy   A technique that uses ancient acupressure points to release tension and increase circulation. Unlike acupuncture, which uses needles, this technique uses gentle but firm finger pressure.

proanthocyanidin   Grape seed extract. It is believed to offer antioxidant protection against heart disease and cancer.

prolotherapy   A soft tissue injection of dextrose or calcium gluconate that produces a local inflammatory reaction, which is intended to promote healing.

ramelteon   The generic name of a sleep agent that is marketed under the brand name Rozerem; it mimics the action of melatonin.

reactive fibromyalgia   A type of fibromyalgia that occurs after sudden trauma.

reflex sympathetic dystrophy (RSD)   Neurological condition, usually affecting an upper or lower extremity after a proximal trauma, which is characterized by pain and vascular irregularity.

REM (rapid eye movement) sleep   The last stage of sleep where, although we remain paralyzed, our brain behaves as if we are awake. This stage allows us to dream.

repetitive transcranial magnetic stimulation (rTMS)   See "transcranial magnetic stimulation."

restless leg syndrome   An overwhelming urge to move the legs as a result of unpleasant or uncomfortable sensations, often leading to difficulty with sleep.

S-adenosyl-methionine (SAM-e)   A nonprescription supplement that may protect certain neurons from damage.

scleroderma   An autoimmune disease associated with thickening of the skin and damage to the lungs, the esophagus, and the vascular system.

scoliosis   Curvature of the spine.

selective serotonin reuptake inhibitor (SSRI)   Several types serve as popular antidepressants.

sensory cortex   The outer part of the brain that interprets the origin or the specific location of the pain message.

serotonin   A neurotransmitter that fosters a sense of satisfaction and plays an important role in mood disorders.

serotonin-norepinephrine reuptake inhibitors (SNRI)   A type of antidepressant that may help to reduce the painful symptoms that sometimes accompany depression.

sertraline   The generic name of a selective serotonin reuptake inhibitor (SSRI) marketed under the brand name Zoloft; an antidepressant.

shiatsu   A type of massage that reaches into deep connective tissue.

Sjögren's syndrome   An inflammatory autoimmune syndrome that affects the salivary and the lacrimal glands, sometimes associated with lupus or rheumatoid disease.

sleep apnea   An airway obstruction that interrupts normal sleep.

sleep spindles   Fast brain waves, 12 to 14 cycles per second, that appear in stage 2 sleep.

sodium oxybate   A synthetic form of GHB (gamma-hydroxybutyrate) that is used in the treatment of narcolepsy and cataplexy.

spinothalamic tract   The pain pathway from the spinal cord to the brain.

splenius   Supportive muscles behind the neck; they help support the weight of the skull.

substance P   A neuropeptide that functions as a neurotransmitter and is involved in the transmission of pain impulses from peripheral receptors to the central nervous system.

sympathectomy   The disruption or the surgical division of sympathetic nerves, usually performed to improve blood flow or reduce pain.

systemic lupus erythematosus   A chronic rheumatic disease that manifests in an overactivity of the immune system and presents with fatigue, joint pain, skin rash, and occasionally organ damage. Also called lupus.

tai chi   An ancient Chinese system of exercise and meditation.

TEDIOUS syndrome   Originally described by David Trock, M.D.; an overlap of pain, fatigue, and obesity, particularly among those with metabolic syndrome or morbid obesity.

temporomandibular joint (TMJ)   A joint that connects the jawbone (mandible) to the skull.

temporalis   A muscle involved in chewing; it is prone to myofascial pain and shortening.

tender points   Specific areas of the body that are particularly sensitive to pressure in a person who has fibromyalgia.

thalamus   A part of the forebrain; it receives and relays neurological information.

theta waves   Brain waves that appear in stage 1 sleep, at about 3 to 7 cycles per second.

thrombophlebitis   Vascular inflammation or obstruction.

tiagabine   An anticonvulsant that is used to partially control seizures.

topiramate   An anticonvulsant.

transcranial magnetic stimulation   The application of a pulsed magnetic field to the brain; it creates microcurrents of electricity that may reduce depression and possibly pain. See also "rTMS."

transcutaneous electrical nerve stimulation (TENS)   A physical therapy modality that is used to disrupt pain impulses to the spinal cord.

trapezius   A muscle on the side of the neck.

tumor necrosis factor (TNF-alpha)   An inflammatory mediator or cytokine; it promotes immune activity.

valerian root   A perennial herb that is used to promote sleep.

ventrolateral preoptic (VLPO) area   The sleep center of the brain.

virtual reality (VR) therapy   A type of therapy that simulates a real situation; it is currently under investigation as a method to relieve pain and emotional distress.

whiplash   A sudden hyperextension-flexion injury to ligaments in the neck.

Xylocaine   A brand name for lidocaine; it is used for anesthesia.

Xyrem   A brand name for the generic drug sodium oxybate, a sleep agent.

zolpidem   The generic name for a sleep agent that is marketed under the brand name Ambien.

REFERENCES

Aaron LA, Burke MM, Buchwald D. Overlapping conditions among patients with chronic fatigue syndrome, fibromyalgia, and temporomandibular disorder. *Arch Intern Med* 2000; 160(2):221–227.

Abbadie C, Brown JL, Mantyh PW, Basbaum AI. Spinal cord substance P receptor immunoreactivity increases in both inflammatory and nerve injury models of persistent pain. *Neuroscience* 1996; 70(1):201–209.

Adler GK, Kinsley BT, Hurwitz S, et al. Reduced hypothalamic-pituitary and sympathoadrenal responses to hypoglycemia in women with fibromyalgia syndrome. *Am J Med* 1999; 106(5):534–543.

Al Allaf AW, Dunbar KL, Hallum NS, et al. A case-control study examining the role of physical trauma in the onset of fibromyalgia syndrome. *Rheumatology* (Oxford) 2002; 41(4):450–453.

Andersen OK, Felsby S, Nicolaisen L, et al. The effect of ketamine on stimulation of primary and secondary hyperalgesic areas induced by capsaicin—a double-blind, placebo-controlled, human experimental study. *Pain* 1996; 66:51–62.

Arendt-Nielsen L, Graven-Nielsen T, Svensson P, Jensen TS. Temporal summation in muscles and referred pain areas: an experimental human study. *Muscle Nerve* 1997; 20(10):1311–1313.

Arnold LM, Hudson JI, Hess EV, et al. Family study of fibromyalgia. *Arthritis Rheum* 2004; 50(3):944–952.

Arroya JF, Cohen ML. Abnormal responses to electrocutaneous stimulation in fibromyalgia. *J Rheumatol* 1993; 20:1925–1931.

Bajaj P, Madsen H, Arendt-Nielsen L. Endometriosis is associated with central sensitization: a psychophysical controlled study. *J Pain* 2003; 4(7):372–380.

Barkhuizen A, Schoeplin GS, Bennett RM. Fibromyalgia: a prominent feature in patients with musculoskeletal problems in chronic hepatitis C: a report of 12 patients. *J Clinical Rheumatology* 1996; 2:180–184.

Bendtsen L, Norregaard J, Jensen R, Olesen J. Evidence of qualitatively altered nociception in patients with fibromyalgia. *Arthritis Rheum* 1997; 40:98–102.

Bennett DL. Neurotrophic factors: important regulators of nociceptive function. *Neuroscientist* 2001; 7(1):13–17.

Bennett RM. Adult growth hormone deficiency in patients with fibromyalgia. *Curr Rheumatol Rep* 2002; 4(4):306–312.

Bennett RM. Fibromyalgia syndrome review. *Journal of Musculoskeletal Pain* 2004; 12(1):35–49.

Bergman S, Herrstrom P, Hogstrom K, et al. Chronic musculoskeletal pain, prevalence rates, and sociodemographic associations in a Swedish population study. *J Rheumatol* 2001; 28(6):1369–1377.

Banic B, Petersen-Felix S, Andersen OK, et al. Evidence for spinal cord hypersensitivity in chronic pain after whiplash injury and in fibromyalgia. *Pain* 2004; 107:7–15.

Bremner JD, Vythilingam M, Anderson G, et al. Assessment of the hypothalamic-pituitary-adrenal axis over a 24-hour diurnal period and in response to neuroendocrine challenges in women with and without childhood sexual abuse and posttraumatic stress disorder. *Biol Psychiatry* 2003; 54(7): 710–718.

Burckhardt CS, O'Reilly CA, Wiens AN, et al. Assessing depression in fibromyalgia patients. *Arthritis Care Res* 1994; 7:35–39.

Buskila D, Neumann L, Hazanov I, Carmi R. Familial aggregation in the fibromyalgia syndrome. *Semin Arthritis Rheum* 1996; 26:605–611.

Buskila D, Neumann L, Vaisberg G, Alkalay D, Wolfe F. Increased rates of fibromyalgia following cervical spine injury. A controlled study of 161 cases of traumatic injury. *Arthritis Rheum* 1997; 40:446–452.

Buskila D, Odes LR, Neumann L, Odes HS. Fibromyalgia in inflammatory bowel disease. *J Rheumatol* 1999; 26(5):1167–1171.

Carmona L, Ballina J, Gabriel R, Laffon A. The burden of musculoskeletal diseases in the general population of Spain: results from a national survey. *Ann Rheum Dis* 2001; 60(11):1040–1045.

Chrousos GP. The hypothalamic-pituitary-adrenal axis and immune-mediated inflammation. *New England Journal of Medicine* 1995; 332: 1351–1362.

Clauw DJ. Fibromyalgia: more than just a musculoskeletal disease. *Am Fam Physician* 1995; 52:843–851, 853–854.

Cohen H, Neumann L, Shore M, et al. Autonomic dysfunction in patients with fibromyalgia: application of power spectral analysis of heart rate variability (see comments). *Semin Arthritis Rheum* 2000; 29(4):217–227.

Cook DB, Lange G, Ciccone DS, et al. Functional imaging of pain in patients with primary fibromyalgia. *J Rheumatol* 2004; 31(2):364–378.

Desmeules JA, Cedraschi C, Rapiti E, et al. Neurophysiologic evidence for a central sensitization in patients with fibromyalgia. *Arthritis Rheum* 2003; 48(5):1420–1429.

Dinerman H, Steere AC. Fibromyalgia following Lyme disease: association with neurologic involvement and lack of response to antibiotic therapy. *Arthritis Rheum* 33(9), S136. 1990. Ref Type: Abstract.

Donaldson MS, Speight N, Loomis S. Fibromyalgia syndrome improved using a mostly raw vegetarian diet: an observational study. *BMC Complement Altern Med.* 2001; 1(1):7. *Epub* 2001 September 26.

Flier JS, Lemquist JK. A good night's sleep: future antidote to the obesity epidemic? *Annals of Internal Medicine* 2004; 141(11):885.

Forseth KO, Gran JT. The prevalence of fibromyalgia among women aged 20–49 years in Arendal, Norway. *Scand J Rheumatol.* 1992; 21:74–78.

Geisser ME, Casey KL, Brucksch CB, et al. Perception of noxious and innocuous heat stimulation among healthy women and women with fibromyalgia: association with mood, somatic focus, and catastrophizing. *Pain* 2003; 102(3):243–250.

Gerra G, Zaimovic A, Giucastro G, et al. Neurotransmitter-hormonal responses to psychological stress in peripubertal subjects: relationship to aggressive behavior. *Life Sci* 1998; 62(7):617–625.

Giovengo SL, Russell IJ, Larsonn AA. Increased concentrations of nerve growth factor in cerebrospinal fluid of patients with fibromyalgia. *J Rheumatol* 1999; 26(7):1564–1569.

Goldman JA. Fibromyalgia and hypermobility. *J Rheumatol* 2001; 28(4): 920–921.

Grady EP, Carpenter MT, Koenig CD, Older SA, Battafarano DF. Rheumatic findings in Gulf War veterans. *Arch Intern Med* 1998; 158(4):367–371.

Gracely RH, Petzke F, Wolf JM, Clauw DJ. Functional magnetic resonance imaging evidence of augmented pain processing in fibromyalgia. *Arthritis Rheum* 2002; 46(5):1333–1343.

Grafe A, Wollina U, Tebbe B, et al. Fibromyalgia in lupus erythematosus. *Acta Derm Venereol* 1999; 79(1):62–64.

Graven-Nielsen T, Aspegren KS, Henriksson KG, et al. Ketamine reduces muscle pain, temporal summation, and referred pain in fibromyalgia patients. *Pain* 2000; 85(3):483–491.

Gur A, Karakoc M, Nas K, et al. Cytokines and depression in cases with fibromyalgia. *J Rheumatol* 2002; 29(2):358–361.

Gursoy S. Absence of association of the serotonin transporter gene polymorphism with the mentally healthy subset of fibromyalgia patients. *Clin Rheumatol* 2002; 21(3):194–197.

Hoffman H, Patterson D. Virtual reality pain distraction. Bulletin, American Pain Society, Spring 2005.

Hoffman HG, Virtual reality therapy. *Scientific American*, August 2004.

Inanici F, Yunus MB. History of fibromyalgia: past to present. *Curr Pain Headache Rep* 2004; 8:369–378.

Johnson K. Fibromyalgia disturbs sensory volume control. *Internal Medicine News*, June 1, 2004; 17.

Kaluta A, Trock D, Burns D, Trock E. A holistic approach to reducing the symptoms of fibromyalgia. *Connecticut Medicine* 1999; 63(8):477.

Kiecolt-Glaser JK, Preacher KJ, MacCallum RC, et al. Chronic stress and age-related increases in the proinflammatory cytokine IL-6. *Proc Natl Acad Sci USA* 2003; 100(15):9090–9095.

King S, Difede J. Firefighter in distress. *New York*, June 13, 2005; 50.

Kivimaki M, Leino-Arjas P, Virtanen M, et al. Work stress and incidence of newly diagnosed fibromyalgia: prospective cohort study. *J Psychosom Res*, November 2004; 57(5):417–422.

Koltzenburg M, Torebjork HE, Wahren LK. Nociceptor modulated central sensitization causes mechanical hyperalgesia in acute chemogenic and chronic neuropathic pain. *Brain* 1994; 117(Pt 3):579–591.

Kosek E, Ekholm J, Hansson P. Sensory dysfunction in fibromyalgia patients with implications for pathogenic mechanisms. *Pain* 1996; 68:375–383.

Kwiatek R, Barnden L, Tedman R, et al. Regional cerebral blood flow in fibromyalgia: single-photon-emission computed tomography evidence of reduction in the pontine tegmentum and thalami. *Arthritis Rheum* 2000; 43(12):2823–2833.

Lam, P. Tai chi. *Arthritis Self-Management*, November/December 2003; 22–32.

Lapossy E, Maleitzke R, Hrycaj P, et al. The frequency of transition of chronic low back pain to fibromyalgia. *Scand J Rheumatol* 1995; 24:29–33.

Lautenbacher S, Rollman GB. Possible deficiencies of pain modulation in fibromyalgia. *Clin J Pain* 1997; 13(3):189–196.

Levine JD, Dardick SJ, Basbaum AI, Scipio E. Reflex neurogenic inflammation. I. Contribution of the peripheral nervous system to spatially remote inflammatory responses that follow injury. *J Neurosci* 1985; 5(5): 1380–1386.

Littlejohn GO. Balanced treatments for fibromyalgia. *Arthritis Rheum*, September 2004; 50(9):2725–2729.

Littlejohn GO, Weinstein C, Helme RD. Increased neurogenic inflammation in fibrositis syndrome. *J Rheumatol* 1987; 14:1022–1025.

Liu Z, Welin M, Bragee B, Nyberg F. A high-recovery extraction procedure for quantitative analysis of substance P and upload peptides in human cerebrospinal fluid. *Peptides* 2000; 21(6):853–860.

Lorenz J, Grasedyck K, Bromm B. Middle and long latency somatosensory evoked potentials after painful laser stimulation in patients with fibromyalgia syndrome. *Electroencephalogry Clin Neurophysiol* 1996; 100:165–168.

Mageri W, Wilk SH, Treede RD. Secondary hyperalgesia and perceptual wind-up following intradermal injection of capsaicin in humans. *Pain* 1998; 74(2–3):257–268.

Mengshoel AM, Heggen K. Recovery from fibromyalgia—previous patients' own experiences. *Disabil Rehabil* 2004; 26(1):46–53.

Mense S. Neurobiological concepts of fibromyalgia—the possible role of descending spinal tracts. *Scand J Rheumatol Suppl* 2000; 113:24–29.

Mense S. The pathogenesis of muscle pain. *Curr Pain Headache Rep* 2003; 7(6):419–425.

Meyer HP. Myofascial pain syndrome and its suggested role in the pathogenesis and treatment of fibromyalgia syndrome. *Curr Pain Headache Rep* 2002; 6(4):274–283.

Mountz JM, Bradley LA, Modell JG, et al. Fibromyalgia in women. Abnormalities of regional cerebral blood flow in the thalamus and the caudate nucleus are associated with low pain threshold levels. *Arthritis Rheum* 1995; 38:926–938.

Naranjo A, Ojeda S, Francisco F, et al. Fibromyalgia in patients with rheumatoid arthritis is associated with higher scores of disability. *Ann Rheum Dis* 2002; 61(7):660–661.

Offenbaecher M, Glatzeder K, Ackenheil M. Self-reported depression, familial history of depression and fibromyalgia (FM), and psychological distress in patients with FM. *J Rheumatol* 1998; 57 Suppl 2:94–96.

Ostuni P, Botsios C, Sfriso P, et al. Fibromyalgia in Italian patients with primary Sjögren's syndrome. *Joint Bone Spine* 2002; 69(1).51–57.

Owens MJ, Nemeroff CB. Role of serotonin in the pathophysiology of depression: focus on the serotonin transporter. *Clin Chem* 1994; 40:288–295.

Perlstein S. Duloxetine benefits women with fibromyalgia, not men. *Internal Medicine News*, June 1, 2004; 17.

Pillemer SR, Bradley LA, Crofford LJ, et al. The neuroscience and endocrinology of fibromyalgia. *Arthritis & Rheumatism* 1997; 40:1928–1939.

Raj SR, Brouillard D, Simpson CS, et al. Dysautonomia among patients with fibromyalgia: a noninvasive assessment. *J Rheumatol* 2000; 27(11): 2660–2665.

Reginato AJ, Falasca GF, Pappu R, et al. Musculoskeletal manifestations of osteomalacia: report of 26 cases and literature review [in process citation]. *Semin Arthritis Rheum* 1999; 28(5):287–304.

Russell IJ. Neurochemicals in fibromyalgia. *The Supplement*, National Fibromyalgia Association, March–June 2004; 6.

Russell IJ, Orr MD, Littman B, et al. Elevated cerebrospinal fluid levels of substance P in patients with the fibromyalgia syndrome. *Arthritis Rheum* 1994; 37(11):1593–1601.

Salemi S, Rethage J, Wollina U, et al. Detection of interleukin 1beta (IL-1beta), IL-6, and tumor necrosis factor-alpha in skin of patients with fibromyalgia. *J Rheumatol* 2003; 30(1):146–150.

Sapolsky RM. *Biology and Human Behavior: The Neurological Origins of Individuality*. Chantilly, VA: Teaching Company, 1998.

Scharf MB, Baumann M, Berkowitz, DV. The effects of sodium oxybate on clinical symptoms and sleep patterns in patients with fibromyalgia. *Journal of Rheumatology* 2003; 30(5):1070–1074.

Simms RW, Ferrante N, Craven DE. High prevalence of fibromyalgia syndrome (FMS) in human immunodeficiency virus type 1 (HIV) infected patients with polyarthralgia. *Arthritis Rheum* 1990; 33(9):S136 (abstract).

Smith JD, Terpening CM, Schmidt SO, et al. Relief of fibromyalgia symptoms following discontinuation of dietary excitotoxins. *Ann Pharmacother*, June 2001; 35(6):702–706.

Sorensen J, Bengtsson A, Backman E, et al. Pain analysis in patients with fibromyalgia: effects of intravenous morphine, lidocaine and ketamine. *Scand J Rheumatol* 1995; 24:360–365.

Sorensen J, Graven-Nielsen T, Henriksson KG, et at. Hyperexcitablity in fibromyalgia. *J Rheumatol* 1998; 25(1):152–155.

Stahl SM. Here today and not gone tomorrow: the curse of chronic pain and other central sensitization syndromes. *J Clin Psychiatry* 2003; 64(8): 863–864.

Staud R, Vierck CJ, Cannon RL, et al. Abnormal sensitization and temporal summation of second pain (wind-up) in patients with fibromyalgia syndrome. *Pain* 2001; 91(1–2):165–175.

Staud R, Cannon RC, Mauderli AP, et al. Temporal summation of pain from mechanical stimulation of muscle tissue in normal controls and subjects with fibromyalgia syndrome. *Pain* 2003; 102(1-2):87–95.

Suhr JA. Neuropsychological impairment in fibromyalgia. Relation to depression, fatigue, and pain. *J Psychosom Res* 2003; 55(4):321–329.

Tucker M. Yoga alleviates fibromyalgia pain, small study shows. *Rheumatology News*, April 2005; 6.

Vgontzas AN, Papanicolaou DA, Bixler EO, et al. Circadian interleukin-6 secretion and quality and depth of sleep. *J Clinical Endocrinology & Metabolism* 1999; 84:2603–2607.

Vgontzas AN, Papanicolaou DA, Bixler EO, et al. Elevation of plasma cytokines in disorders of excessive daytime sleepiness: role of sleep disturbance and obesity. *J Clin Endocrinol Metab* 1997; 82:1313–1316.

Volpato S, Guralnik JM, Ferrucci L, et al. Cardiovascular disease, interleukin-6, and risk of mortality in older women: the women's health and aging study. *Circulation* 2001; 520;103(7):947–953.

Wallace DJ, Linker-Israeli M, Hallegua D, et al. Cytokines play an aetiopathogenetic role in fibromyalgia: a hypothesis and pilot study. *Rheumatology* (Oxford) 2001; 40(7):743–749.

Watkins LR, Maier SF. Glia: a novel drug discovery target for clinical pain. *Nature Reviews/Drug Discovery*, December 2003; 2:973–985.

White KP, Thompson J. Fibromyalgia syndrome in an Amish community: a controlled study to determine disease and symptom prevalence. *J Rheumatol* 2003; 30(8):1835–1840.

Wolfe F, Ross K, Anderson J, et al. The prevalence and characteristics of fibromyalgia in the general population. *Arthritis Rheum* 1995; 38: 19–28.

Wolfe F, Smythe HA, Yunus MB, et al. The American College of Rheumatology 1990 criteria for the classification of fibromyalgia: Report of the Multicenter Criteria Committee. *Arthritis Rheum* 1990; 33:160–172.

Wood, PB. Stress and dopamine: implications for the pathophysiology of chronic widespread pain. *Medical Hypotheses* 2004; 62:420–424.

Woolf CJ. Pain: moving from symptom control toward mechanism-specific pharmacologic management. *Annals of Internal Medicine* 2004; 140: 441–451.

Yunus MB. Psychological aspects of fibromyalgia syndrome: a component of the dysfunctional spectrum syndrome. *Baillieres Clin Rheumatol* 1994; 8:811–837.

Yunus, MB. Suffering, science and sabotage. *Journal of Musculoskeletal Pain* 2004; 12(2).

INDEX

ABOUT THE AUTHORS

Dr. David Trock is the chief of rheumatology at Danbury Hospital in Connecticut and an assistant clinical professor of medicine at Yale University School of Medicine. He is board-certified in rheumatology, a fellow of the American College of Physicians, and a noted author and lecturer in the field of arthritis care.

Frances Chamberlain has coauthored books on psychology, biology, and earth science; is a published poet and essayist; teaches composition and communications; and has led creative writing groups and workshops throughout New England for the last twenty years.

Never Cry Wolf